THE DASH DIET RECIPES

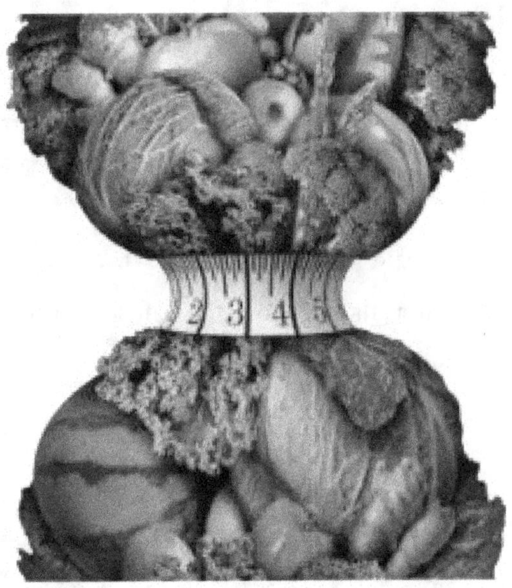

The ultimate guide to delicious low sodium recipes for beginners

Esther James

Copyright © [2023] [Esther James]

All rights reserved.

No part of this book may be reproduced, scanned, or distributed in any printed or electronic form without permission.

Please do not participate in or encourage piracy of copyrighted materials in violation of the author's rights. Purchase only authorized editions.

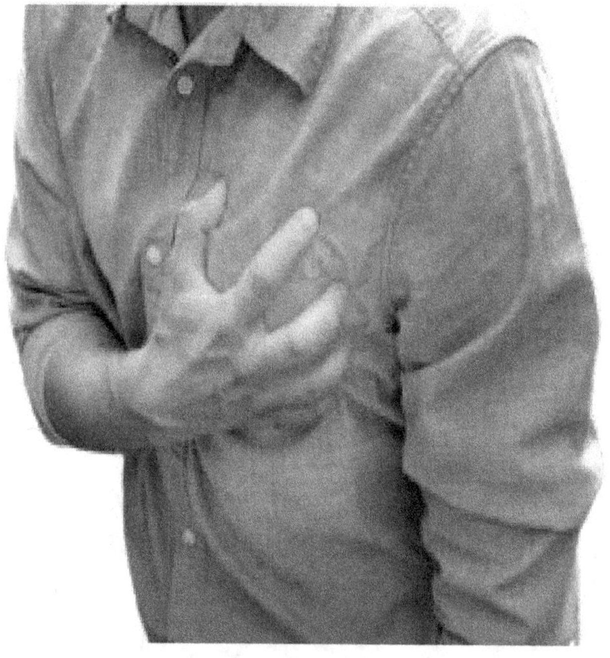

Table of Content

CHAPTER 7 ....**81**

INTRODUCTION

Once upon a time, there was a woman named Jane who had always struggled with her weight and being fit. She frequently found herself indulging in unhealthy meals and making poor dietary choices.

Jane decided one day that enough was enough and she was determined to make a difference. She knew she needed to change her eating habits, but she didn't know where to begin. She stumbled upon The Big Dash Diet Cookbook for Beginners Low Sodium Recipes at that time. She was drawn in by the promise of delicious and healthful low-sodium dishes that would aid her in her quest for a better lifestyle.

Jane decided to give it a shot and purchased the cookbook. She quickly flicked through the pages when it came, astounded by the range of dishes offered. There was something for everyone, from breakfast to dinner and everything in between.

Jane began by experimenting with some of the morning dishes, such as the Blueberry Oatmeal and the Vegetable and Egg Breakfast Sandwich. She was pleasantly pleased by how tasty they were, and she felt satiated and energy all day.

Jane discovered a whole new world of healthy food as she proceeded to peruse the cookbook. She tried new veggies and fruits, learned to cook using low-sodium herbs and spices, and discovered new methods to make her favorite foods without compromising flavor.

Jane saw a considerable improvement in her health and well-being over time. She felt more energetic, more secure in her body, and even saw improvements in her complexion and hair.

Her friends and family were astounded by her change and inquired as to her secret. Jane enthusiastically handed them The Big Dash Diet Cookbook for Beginners Low Sodium Recipes, encouraging them to give it a try.

Jane was able to establish a healthy and sustainable way of eating that she loved thanks to the cookbook. She used the cookbook for years, experimenting with different dishes and learning new ways to live a healthy and happy life.

If you want to enhance your health and lower your sodium intake, The Big Dash Diet Cookbook for Beginners Low Sodium Recipes is the book for you.

This cookbook will help you through the process of making tasty, low-sodium foods that are simple to prepare and good for your health.

You'll learn the fundamentals of low-sodium cooking as well as how to incorporate it into your everyday diet. You will also get access to lots of low sodium and flavorful recipes.

The Big Dash Diet Cookbook for Beginners Low Sodium Recipes is great for anyone who wish to cut their salt consumption without compromising flavor. These dishes are simply adaptable to your diet and lifestyle requirements.

This cookbook includes useful suggestions and methods for preparing and cooking low-sodium meals, in addition to the recipes.

There are additional recipes for individuals on a low-sodium diet, as well as meals for vegetarians and those who are lactose intolerant.

This cookbook not only teaches you how to create great low sodium meals, but it also pushes you to consider how you may utilize your diet to enhance your overall health.

You'll discover how to make better choices and include whole foods into your diet. You will also learn how to decrease your salt consumption without sacrificing flavor.

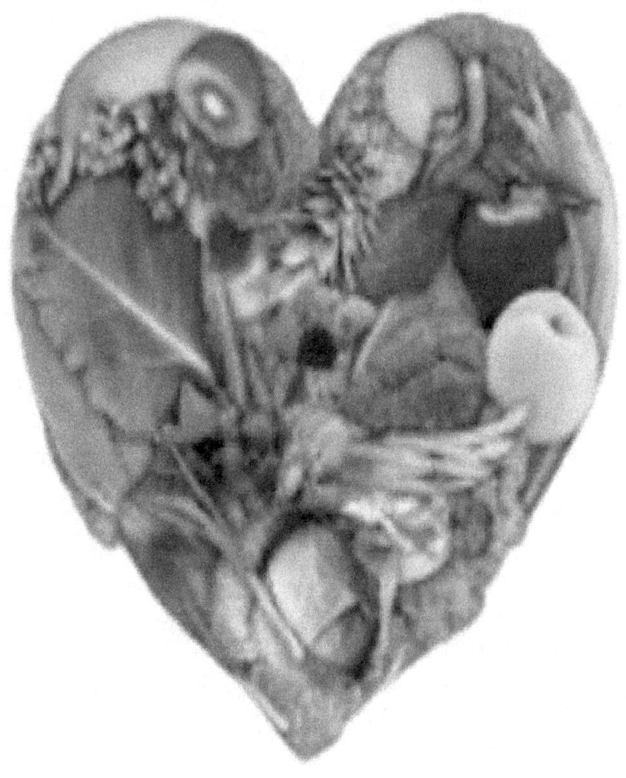

CHAPTER 1

What is Dash Diet?

The DASH diet (Dietary Approaches to Stop Hypertension) is a dietary pattern recommended by the National Institutes of Health (NIH) in the United States to help prevent and treat hypertension (high blood pressure). It emphasizes nutrient-dense foods while limiting sodium, saturated fat, and added sugar consumption.

The DASH diet is rich in fruits, vegetables, low-fat dairy products, whole grains, fish, poultry, beans, seeds, and nuts. It also includes reduced amounts of red meat, sweets, and sugary beverages.

The DASH diet emphasizes portion control and being mindful of what you eat. It also encourages physical activity and a balanced lifestyle.

What is Low Sodium Eating?

Low-sodium eating is a diet that limits the amount of sodium (salt) consumed. This type of diet is recommended for people with high blood pressure, heart failure, and other medical conditions. Eating less sodium can help reduce blood pressure and the risk of heart disease and stroke.

Low-sodium eating usually consists of avoiding processed foods and eating more fresh fruits, vegetables, and whole grains.

In addition to limiting sodium, it is also important to eat a balanced diet that includes plenty of fiber, lean proteins, and healthy fats. Avoiding excessive amounts of saturated fats, sugar, and processed foods is also recommended.

People on a low-sodium diet should also limit their alcohol intake and exercise regularly. Low-sodium eating can help improve heart health and reduce the risk of stroke, heart attack, and other health problems.

Benefits of Low Sodium Eating

Low sodium eating has a variety of potential health benefits which includes the followings:

1. Reduced Risk of High Blood Pressure: Low-sodium diets can reduce the risk of high blood pressure, which is a major risk factor for heart disease, stroke and kidney disease.

2. Improved Heart Health: Reducing the amount of sodium you eat can also help reduce your risk of heart disease.

3. **Increased Energy Levels**: Eating a low-sodium diet can help you maintain your energy levels throughout the day.

4. **Reduced Risk of Kidney Disease:** Eating a low-sodium diet can help reduce the risk of kidney disease.

5. Improved Digestion: Low-sodium diets can help improve digestion and reduce the risk of gastrointestinal problems.

6. Weight Loss: Eating a low-sodium diet can help you lose weight, as it helps to reduce water retention and bloating.

7. **Reduced Bloating:** Eating a low-sodium diet can reduce bloating and water retention, which can help you feel more comfortable.

8. Improved Hydration: Eating a low-sodium diet can help improve hydration, which is important for overall health.

9. Improved Detoxification: Eating a low-sodium diet can help improve detoxification, as it helps to remove excess sodium from the body.

10. Reduced Risk of Cancer: Eating a low-sodium diet can help reduce the risk of certain types of cancer, such as stomach and colorectal cancer.

11. Improved Cognitive Function: Eating a low-sodium diet can help improve cognitive function, as it helps to reduce inflammation in the brain.

12. Improved Skin Health: Eating a low-sodium diet can help improve skin health, as it helps to reduce the risk of acne and other skin problems.

13. Improved Mood: Eating a low-sodium diet can help improve mood, as it helps to reduce stress and anxiety.

14. Reduced Risk of Diabetes: Eating a low-sodium diet can also help reduce the risk of type 2 diabetes.

15. Improved Kidney Health: Eating a low-sodium diet can help improve kidney health, as it helps to reduce the risk of kidney stones.

16. Reduced Risk of Stroke: Eating a low-sodium diet can also help reduce the risk of stroke.

17. Reduced Risk of Alzheimer's: Eating a low-sodium diet can also help reduce the risk of Alzheimer's disease.

Getting Started with the Big Dash Diet

The Big Dash Diet is a healthy eating plan that focuses on reducing the amount of processed foods and eating more nutrient-dense, whole foods.

Here are some tips to get you started:

1. **Begin with a plan.** The Big Dash Diet recommends making a weekly diet plan that includes three meals and two snacks per day. This will assist you in staying on track and consuming the proper foods.

2. **Include a variety of fruits and veggies**. Fruits and vegetables are essential components of the Big Dash Diet and should comprise the majority of your meals. Aim for at least five servings of fruits and vegetables per day.

3. **Choose lean proteins.** Lean proteins like chicken, fish, and beans are essential for supplying your body with the nutrition it requires. Include a lean protein at least once every day.

 4. **Reduce your intake of processed and artificial foods.** Processed and artificial foods contain harmful ingredients

and are not permitted on the Big Dash Diet. Avoid eating these meals as much as possible.

5. Include healthy fats. The Big Dash Diet emphasizes healthy fats like olive oil, avocados, and almonds. Make healthy fats a regular part of your diet.

6. Consume plenty of water. It is critical for your health to stay hydrated. Drink at least eight glasses of water per day.

7. Exercise frequently. Exercise is a crucial component of living a healthy lifestyle and getting the most out of the Big Dash Diet. Every day, aim for at least 30 minutes of exercise.

By following these guidelines, you can begin the Big Dash Diet and begin feeling healthier and more energized.

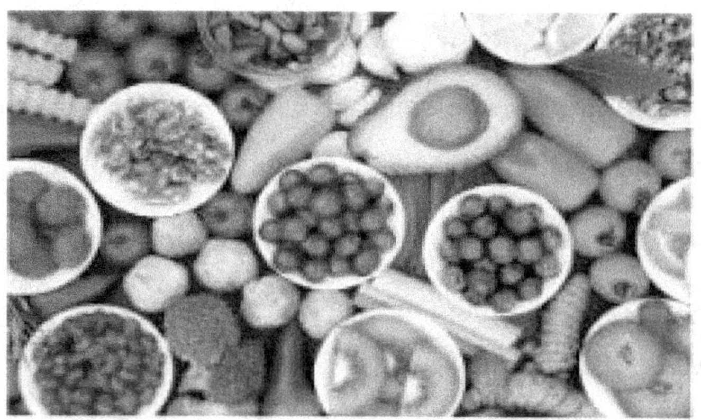

CHAPTER 2

Understanding Low Sodium Diets

A low-sodium diet restricts the quantity of sodium and salt intake. The average American eats more than 3,400 milligrams of sodium per day, significantly exceeding the recommended daily limit of 2,300 milligrams.

A low-sodium diet restricts sodium consumption to 1,500 mg or less per day. This diet can help lower the risk of hypertension, stroke, and heart disease. It also aids in the reduction of boating and water retention.

Processed meals, canned soups, processed meats, frozen dinners, and fast food are all examples of high-sodium foods to avoid on a low-sodium diet. Eating fresh foods and preparing at home can help you consume less sodium.

Reducing salt and replacing it with herbs, spices, and other flavorings can also help reduce sodium intake. Canned veggies, pickles, olives, and salted nuts and seeds are also high in sodium.

When shopping, it is critical to study nutrition labels and select foods low in salt. Several items have low-sodium alternatives, such as low-sodium versions of canned soups and frozen dinners. It is also critical to request no extra salt when dining out.

A low-sodium diet can help reduce the risk of hypertension, stroke, and heart disease. It can also aid with bloating and water retention.

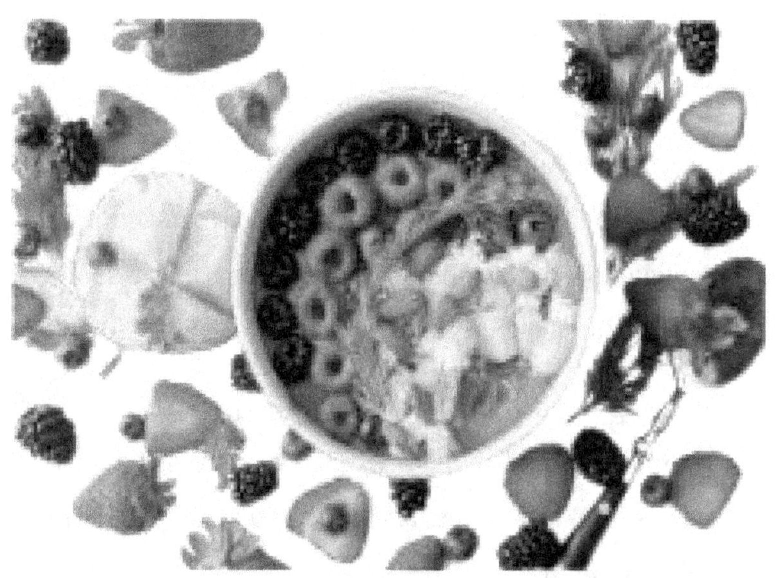

Shopping list

If you're planning to follow the DASH diet and incorporate low-sodium recipes into your meal plan, here's a shopping list that can help you get started:

Fruits and Vegetables

Apples, Bananas, Berries (strawberries, blueberries, raspberries, etc.), Oranges, Grapefruit, Pineapple, Mango

Grapes, Tomatoes, Carrots, Cucumbers, Broccoli, Cauliflower, Spinach, Kale, Brussels sprouts

Sweet potatoes, Squash (zucchini, butternut, etc.)

Bell peppers, Onions, Garlic.

Grains and Starches

Brown rice, Whole wheat pasta, Whole grain bread

Quinoa, Oats, Sweet potatoes, Potatoes,

Protein

Chicken breast (skinless), Turkey breast (skinless)

Fish (salmon, tuna, tilapia, etc.)

Shrimp, Lean beef (round, sirloin, etc.)

Tofu, Beans (black beans, kidney beans, etc.), Lentils

Dairy

Low-fat milk, Low-fat yogurt, Low-fat cheese

Condiments and Spices, Olive oil, Canola oil

Balsamic vinegar, Mustard, Salsa, Hot sauce

Cinnamon, Garlic powder, Onion powder

Salt-free seasoning blends

Remember, when following the DASH diet, it's important to choose low-sodium options whenever possible. Be sure to read food labels carefully and avoid processed and packaged foods that are high in sodium. With this shopping list and a little creativity, you can create delicious and healthy low-sodium meals that will support your overall health and well-being.

CHAPTER 3

30 Days Meal Planning

Day 1:

Oatmeal with berries and walnuts for breakfast

Grilled salmon with steamed veggies for lunch

Curry with chickpeas and spinach for dinner

Day 2:

Smoothie with banana, almond milk, and peanut butter for breakfast

Quinoa Salad with tomatoes, cucumbers, and feta cheese for lunch

Roasted vegetables with grilled chicken for dinner

Day 3:

Breakfast with avocado toast with a poached egg

Baked Sweet Potato with Black Beans and Salsa for Lunch

Dinner: Stir-Fry Veggies with Tofu

Day 4:

Breakfast of an egg white omelet with spinach and mushrooms

Sandwich for lunch: turkey wrap with lettuce and tomato

Fish with roasted broccoli for dinner

Day 5:

Greek yogurt with blueberries and almonds for breakfast

Lentil Soup with Kale and Carrots for Lunch

Grilled chicken with roasted asparagus for dinner

Day 6:

Overnight oats with chia seeds and almond milk for breakfast

Quinoa Salad with black beans, tomatoes, and feta cheese for lunch

Dinner: Tilapia baked with roasted veggies

Day 7:

Smoothie bowl with banana, almond milk, and peanut butter for breakfast

Lentil Soup with Kale and Carrots for Lunch

Vegetarian Burger with Sweet Potato Fries for Dinner

Day 8:

Breakfast of avocado toast and poached egg

Grilled chicken with roasted veggies for lunch

Baked salmon with steamed vegetables for dinner

Day 9:

Oatmeal with berries and walnuts for breakfast

Sandwich for lunch: turkey wrap with lettuce and tomato

Curry with chickpeas and spinach for dinner

Day 10:

Breakfast of an egg white omelet with spinach and mushrooms

Quinoa Salad with tomatoes, cucumbers, and feta cheese for lunch

Roasted vegetables with grilled chicken for dinner

Day 11:

Greek yogurt with blueberries and almonds for breakfast

Baked Sweet Potato with Black Beans and Salsa for Lunch

Dinner: Stir-Fry Veggies with Tofu

Day 12:

Overnight oats with chia seeds and almond milk for breakfast

Lentil Soup with Kale and Carrots for Lunch

Grilled chicken with roasted asparagus for dinner

Day 13:

Smoothie with banana, almond milk, and peanut butter for breakfast

Quinoa Salad with black beans, tomatoes, and feta cheese for lunch

Dinner: Tilapia baked with roasted veggies

Day 14:

Avocado toast with a poached egg for breakfast

Grilled chicken with roasted veggies for lunch

Baked salmon with steamed vegetables for dinner

Day 15:

Oatmeal with berries and walnuts for breakfast

Sandwich for lunch: turkey wrap with lettuce and tomato

Curry with chickpeas and spinach for dinner

Day 16:

Egg white omelet with spinach and mushrooms for breakfast

Quinoa Salad with tomatoes, cucumbers, and feta cheese for lunch

Roasted vegetables with grilled chicken for dinner

Day 17:

Greek yogurt with blueberries and almonds for breakfast

Baked Sweet Potato with Black Beans and Salsa for Lunch

Dinner: Stir-Fry Veggies with Tofu

Day 18:

 Breakfast: Chia seed overnight oats with almond milk

Lentil Soup with Kale and Carrots for Lunch

Grilled chicken with roasted asparagus for dinner

Day 19:

Smoothie with banana, almond milk, and peanut butter for breakfast

Quinoa Salad with black beans, tomatoes, and feta cheese for lunch

Dinner: Tilapia baked with roasted veggies

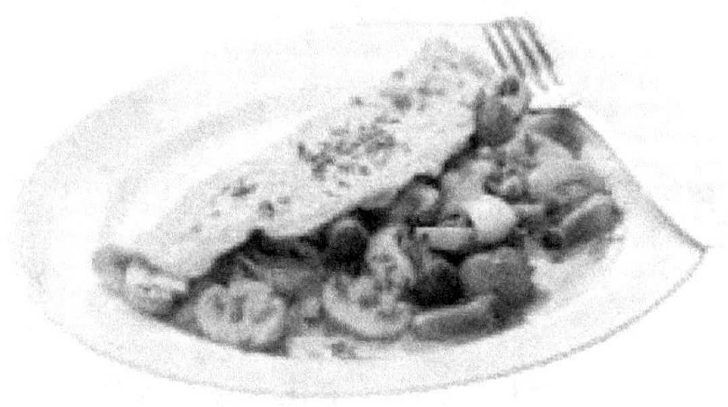

Egg white omelet with spinach and mushroom

Day 20:

 Avocado toast with a poached egg for breakfast

Grilled chicken with roasted veggies for lunch

Baked salmon with steamed vegetables for dinner

Day 21:

Oatmeal with berries and walnuts for breakfast

Sandwich for lunch: turkey wrap with lettuce and tomato

Curry with chickpeas and spinach for dinner

Day 22:

Egg white omelet with spinach and mushrooms for breakfast

Quinoa Salad with tomatoes, cucumbers, and feta cheese for
lunch

Roasted vegetables with grilled chicken for dinner

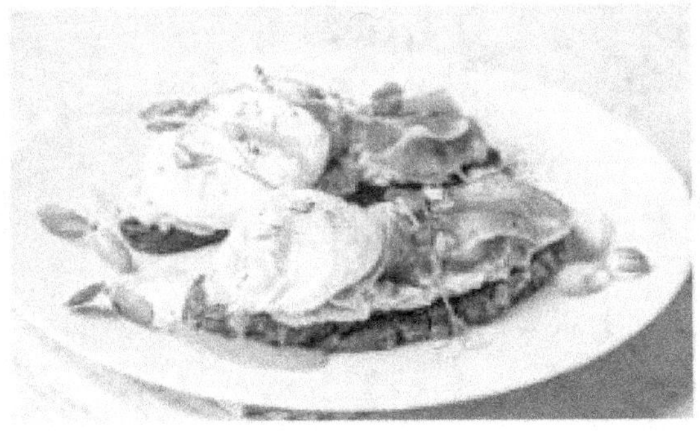

Avocado toast with poached egg

Day 23:

Greek yogurt with blueberries and almonds for breakfast

Baked Sweet Potato with Black Beans and Salsa for Lunch

Dinner: Stir-Fry Veggies with Tofu

Day 24:

Overnight oats with chia seeds and almond milk for breakfast

Lentil Soup with Kale and Carrots for Lunch

Grilled chicken with roasted asparagus for dinner

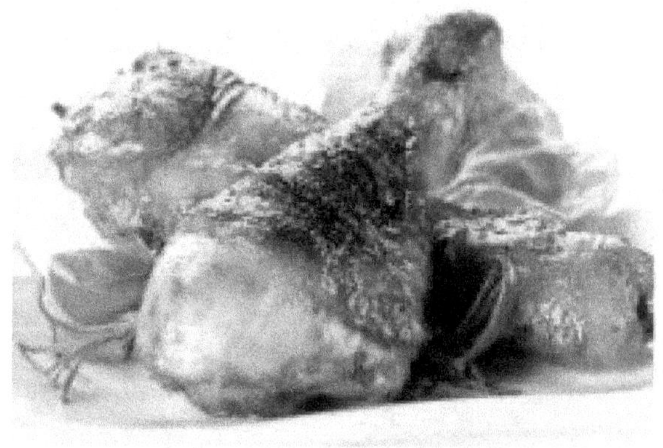

Grilled Chicken with roasted asparagus

Day 25:

Smoothie with banana, almond milk, and peanut butter for breakfast

Quinoa Salad with black beans, tomatoes, and feta cheese for lunch

Dinner: Tilapia baked with roasted veggies

Day 26:

Avocado toast with a poached egg for breakfast

Grilled chicken with roasted veggies for lunch

Baked salmon with steamed vegetables for dinner

Day 27:

 Oatmeal with berries and walnuts for breakfast

Sandwich for lunch: turkey wrap with lettuce and tomato

Curry with chickpeas and spinach for dinner

Day 28:

Egg white omelet with spinach and mushrooms for breakfast
Quinoa Salad with tomatoes, cucumbers, and feta cheese for lunch

Roasted vegetables with grilled chicken for dinner

Day 29:

Greek yogurt with blueberries and almonds for breakfast

Baked Sweet Potato with Black Beans and Salsa for Lunch

Dinner: Stir-Fry Veggies with Tofu

Day 30:

 Overnight oats with chia seeds and almond milk for breakfast

Lentil Soup with Kale and Carrots for Lunch

Grilled chicken with roasted asparagus for dinner

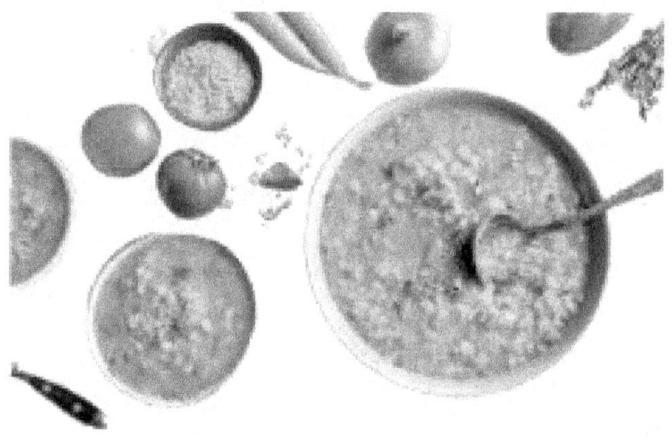

Lentil Soup with kale and carrots

CHAPTER 4

Breakfast Recipes with Preparation method

French toast:

Ingredients:

-4 slices of white bread

-2 eggs, 1/4 cup of milk,

-1 teaspoon of sugar,

-1/4 teaspoon of ground cinnamon,

-1/4 teaspoon of vanilla extract, butter for cooking.

Preparation:

1. In a shallow dish, whisk together the eggs, milk, sugar, cinnamon, and vanilla.

2. In a saucepan with a medium heat, melting the butter.

3. Coat each side of the bread pieces with the egg mixture.

4. Put the slices in the skillet and cook until golden brown on both sides.

5. Garnish with syrup, powdered sugar, and fresh fruit if desired.

Overnight Oats:

Ingredients:

-1/2 cup of oats,

-1/2 cup of milk,

-1/2 cup of plain Greek yogurt,

-1 teaspoon of honey,

- 1/4 teaspoon of ground cinnamon,

-1/4 cup of chopped nuts,

-1/4 cup of dried fruit.

Preparation:

1. In a jar or bowl, combine the oats, milk, yogurt, honey, and cinnamon.

2. Mix together until combined.

3. Cover and place in the refrigerator overnight.

4. In the morning, stir in the nuts and dried fruit. Serve chilled.

Egg and Cheese Sandwich:

Ingredients:

-2 slices of bread,

- 1 egg, 1 slice of cheese,

- 1 tablespoon of butter.

Preparation:

1. In a medium skillet over medium heat, melt the butter.

2. Put the cracked egg into the skillet and cook until done to your liking.

3. Put the cheese on one slice of bread and top with the egg.

4. Put the second slice of bread on top and lightly press down.

5. Fry the sandwich in the skillet until both sides are golden brown.

Serve warm.

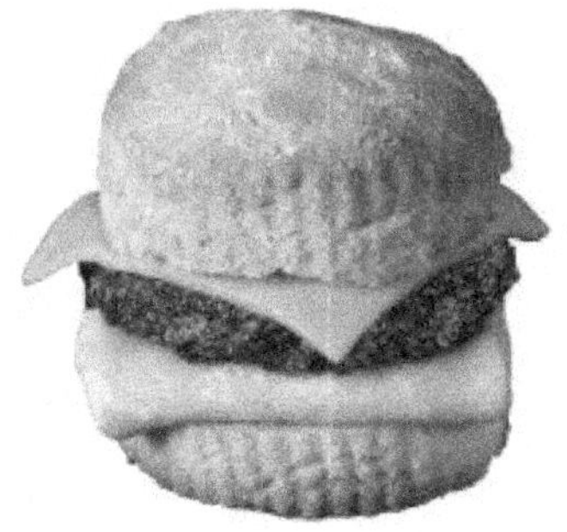

Breakfast Burrito

Ingredients:

-1 flour tortilla,

-2 eggs,

-1/4 cup of shredded cheese,

- 1/4 cup of diced tomatoes,

-1/4 cup of diced onions,

- 1 tablespoon of olive oil, salt and pepper.

Preparation:

In a pan with a medium heat, heat the olive oil.

2. Add the eggs and scramble until done.

3. Add the tomatoes, onions, salt, and pepper, and cook for an additional 2 minutes.

4. Place the egg mixture onto the tortilla and top with the cheese.

5. Roll up the burrito and serve.

Breakfast Quesadilla:

Ingredients:

-2 flour tortillas,

-1/2 cup of shredded cheese,

-1/4 cup of diced tomatoes,

-1/4 cup of diced onions,

-1 tablespoon of butter, salt and pepper.

Preparation:

1. In a medium skillet over medium heat, melt the butter.

2. On the skillet, place one of the tortillas and top with the cheese, tomatoes, and onions.

3. Put the remaining tortilla on top.

4. Cook until the cheese has melted and the crust has turned golden brown.

5. Cut into wedges before serving.

Avocado Toast:

Ingredients:

-2 slices of bread,

-1/2 an avocado,

-1/4 teaspoon of garlic powder

Preparation:

1. Toast the bread until lightly golden brown.

2. Mash the avocado in a bowl and mix in the garlic powder.

3. Spread the avocado mixture onto the toast and serve.

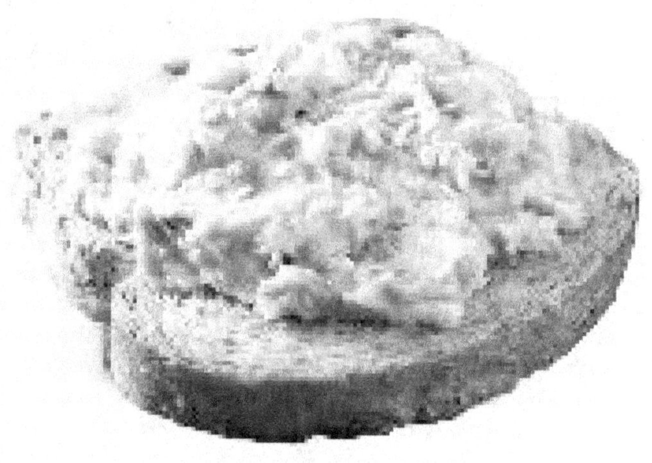

Smoothie Bowl:

Ingredients:

-1 banana,

-1/2 cup of frozen berries,

-1/4 cup of Greek yogurt,

-1/4 cup of almond milk,

-1 teaspoon of honey,

-1/4 cup of granola,

-1/4 cup of fresh fruit.

Preparation:

1. Place the banana, frozen berries, yogurt, almond milk, and honey in a blender and blend until smooth.

2. Pour the mixture into a bowl and top with the granola and fresh fruit. Serve chilled.

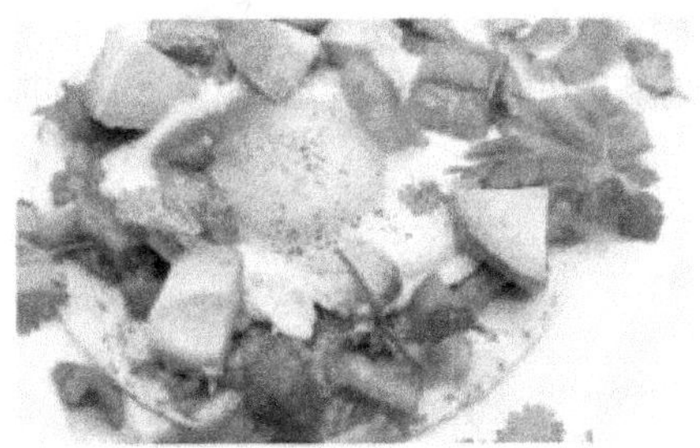

Breakfast Tacos:

Ingredients:

-2 flour tortillas,

-2 eggs,

-1/4 cup of shredded cheese,

-1/4 cup of diced tomatoes,

-1/4 cup of diced onions,

-1 1 tbsp. of olive oil, along with pepper and salt.

Preparation:

1. In a medium skillet over medium heat, melt the butter.

2. Add the eggs and scramble until done.

3. Add the tomatoes, onions, salt, and pepper and cook for an additional 2 minutes.

4. Place the eggs onto the tortillas and top with the cheese. Roll up the tacos and serve.

Huevos Rancheros:

Ingredients:

-2 corn tortillas,

-2 eggs,

-1/4 cup of enchilada sauce,

-1/4 cup of shredded cheese,

-1/4 cup of diced onions,

-1 tablespoon of olive oil, pepper and salt.

Preparation:

Prepare the butter by melting it in a medium skillet over medium heat.

2. Add the eggs and scramble until done.

3. Add the onions, salt, and pepper and cook for an additional 2 minutes.

4. Place the eggs onto the tortillas and top with the enchilada sauce and cheese. Serve.

Biscuits and Gravy:

Ingredients:

-4 biscuits,

-1/2 pound of sausage,

-2 tablespoons of butter,

-2 tablespoons of all-purpose flour,

-1 cup of milk,

-1/2 teaspoon of ground black pepper,

-1/2 teaspoon of garlic powder.

Preparation:

1. Heat a skillet over medium heat and cook the sausage until browned.

2. Set the sausage aside after removing it from the skillet.

3. In the same skillet, melt the butter and add the flour, stirring until combined.

4. Slowly add the milk, stirring constantly until thickened. Add the cooked sausage, pepper, and garlic powder.

Serve over the biscuits.

Oatmeal:

Ingredients:

-1/2 cup of oats,

-1 cup of milk,

-1 tablespoon of honey,

- 1/4 teaspoon of ground cinnamon.

Preparation:

1. In a saucepan, bring the oats and milk to a boil over medium heat.

2. Lower the heat to low and cook for 5 minutes, stirring frequently.

3. Remove from heat and stir in the honey and cinnamon. Serve warm with fresh fruit, nuts, and extra honey.

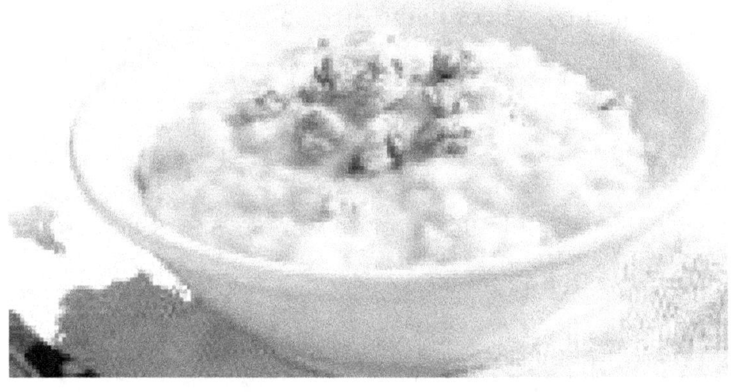

Breakfast Casserole:

Ingredients:

- 8 slices of white bread,

-8 eggs,

-2 cups of milk,

-1 teaspoon of ground mustard,

-1/2 teaspoon of salt,

-1/4 teaspoon of ground black pepper,

-1/2 cup of shredded cheese.

Preparation:

1. Preheat the oven to 375 degrees. Grease a 9x13 inch baking dish.

2. Place the bread slices in the dish and set aside.

3. Whisk together the eggs, milk, mustard, salt, and pepper in a mixing dish.

4. Pour the egg mixture over the bread and top with the cheese. Bake for 45 minutes.

5. Serve warm.

Breakfast Sandwich:

Ingredients:

-2 slices of bread,

- 2 eggs,

-1 slice of cheese,

-1 tablespoon of butter.

Preparation:

1. The butter should be melted in a pan over medium heat.

2. Put the eggs into the skillet and cook until done to preference.

4. Top one slice of bread with the cheese and the egg.

5. Put the other slice of bread on top and lightly press down.

6. In a skillet, cook the sandwich until both sides are golden brown.

Serve hot.

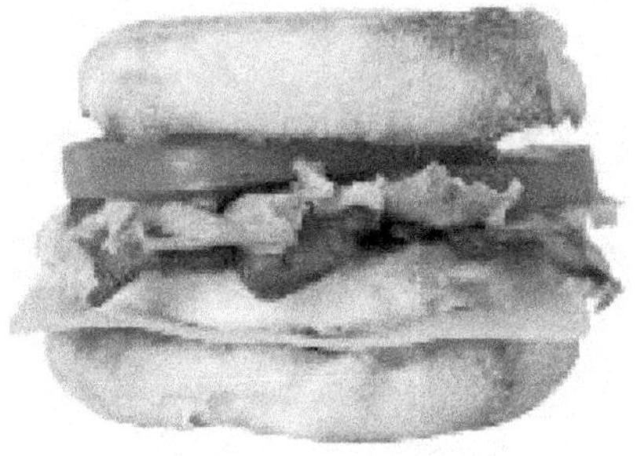

Egg Muffins:

Ingredients:

-6 eggs,

-1/2 cup of diced ham,

-1/4 cup of shredded cheese,

-1/4 cup of diced tomatoes,

- 1/4 cup of diced onions,

-1 tablespoon of olive oil, along with pepper and salt.

Preparation:

Preheat the oven to 375 degrees.

1. Grease a 12-cup muffin tin.

2. Heat the olive oil in a skillet over medium heat.

3. Add the eggs and scramble until done.

4. Add the ham, tomatoes, onions, salt, and pepper, and cook for an additional 2 minutes.

5. Place the eggs into the muffin tin and top with the cheese.

6. Bake for 15 minutes.

7. Serve warm.

CHAPTER 5

Lunch Recipes Preparation

Grilled Chicken and Avocado Salad

Ingredients:

- 2 boneless, skinless chicken breasts

- 2 tablespoons olive oil

- 2 tablespoons lemon juice

- 4 cups mixed greens

- 1 cup cherry tomatoes, halved

- 1/2 cup sliced cucumber

- 1/2 cup sliced avocado

- 2 tablespoons crumbled feta cheese

- Salt and pepper, to taste

Method:

1. Preheat the grill to medium-high heat.

2. Combine the olive oil and lemon juice in a mixing bowl

3. Rub the mixture over the chicken breasts and season with salt and pepper.

4. Place the chicken on the preheated grill and cook for 4-6 minutes per side, until cooked through.

5. Remove the chicken from the grill and let cool before slicing into cubes.

6. In a large bowl, combine the mixed greens, cherry tomatoes, cucumber, avocado, and feta cheese.

7. Toss with the cooled chicken cubes.

8. Sprinkle with olive oil and lemon juice, to taste, then season with salt and pepper.

9. Serve and enjoy.

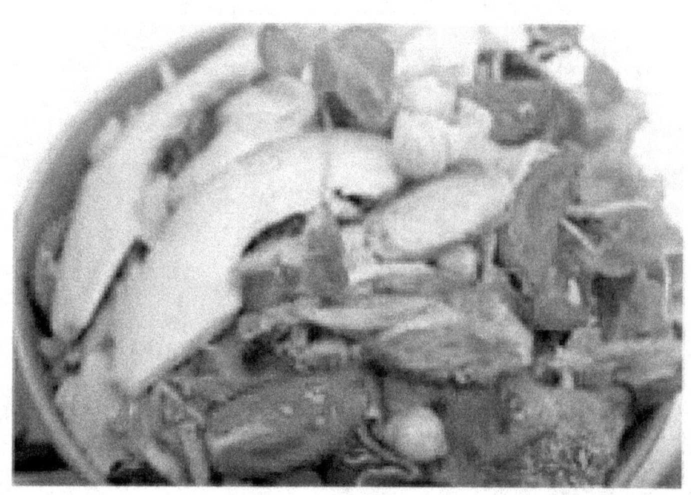

Grilled Chicken and Avocado Salad

Baked Salmon with Spinach and Tomatoes

Ingredients:

- 4 (4-ounce) salmon fillets

- 2 tablespoons olive oil

- 2 cloves garlic, minced

- 2 cups fresh spinach

- 1 cup cherry tomatoes, halved

- 1/4 teaspoon dried oregano

- *Salt and pepper, to taste*

Method:

1. Preheat the oven to 400°F.

2. Line a baking sheet with aluminum foil and coat lightly with nonstick spray.

3. Place the salmon fillets on the baking sheet and brush with olive oil.

4. Top with garlic, spinach, tomatoes, oregano, salt, and pepper.

5. Bake for 15-20 minutes, or until the salmon is thoroughly cooked.

6. Serve and enjoy.

Quinoa Bowl with Black Beans and Corn

Ingredients:

- 1 cup cooked quinoa

- 1/2 cup cooked black beans

- 1/2 cup cooked corn

- 2 tablespoons olive oil

- 2 tablespoons lime juice

- 1/4 teaspoon cumin

- Salt and pepper, to taste

- 2 tablespoons chopped fresh cilantro

Method:

1. In a large bowl, combine the quinoa, black beans, and corn.

2. Drizzle with olive oil and lime juice and season with cumin, salt, and pepper.

3. Toss to combine.

4. Sprinkle with cilantro and serve.

Broccoli and Shrimp Stir Fry

Ingredients:

- 2 tablespoons olive oil

- 1/2 pound shrimp, peeled and deveined

- 1 cup broccoli florets

- 1/2 cup sliced bell pepper

- 2 cloves garlic, minced

- 2 tablespoons reduced-sodium soy sauce

- 1 tablespoon sesame oil

- Salt and pepper, to taste

Method:

1. In a big skillet with a medium-high temperature, heat the olive oil.

2. Add the shrimp and Cook for 2-3 minutes, or until the shrimp are pink and cooked through.

3. Add the broccoli, bell pepper, and garlic and cook for an additional 3-4 minutes.

4. Add the soy sauce and sesame oil and season with salt and pepper.

5. Cook for an additional 1-2 minutes, until everything is cooked through.

6. Serve and enjoy.

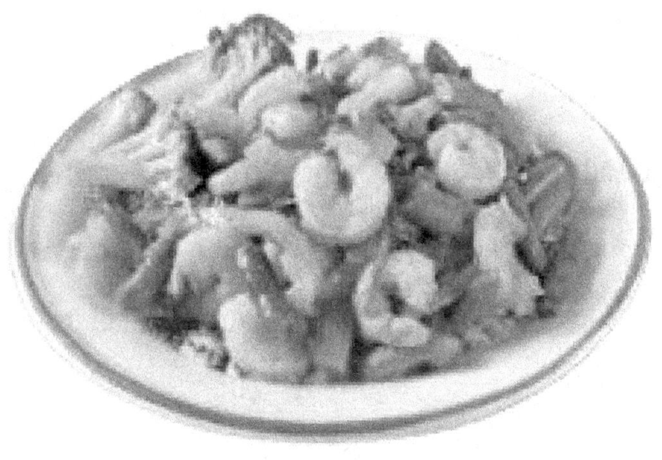

Broccoli and Shrimp Stir Fry

Turkey Burger

Ingredients:

- 1 pound ground turkey

- 2 cloves garlic, minced

- 1/4 teaspoon dried oregano

- 1/4 teaspoon dried basil

- 1/4 teaspoon dried thyme

- 1/4 teaspoon paprika

- Salt and pepper, to taste

- 4 whole-wheat buns

- Lettuce, tomato, and onion, for serving

Method:

1. In a large bowl, combine the ground turkey, garlic, oregano, basil, thyme, paprika, salt, and pepper.

2. Form the mixture into 4 patties.

3. Heat a large skillet over medium-high heat and cook the patties for 4-5 minutes per side, until cooked through.

5. Place the patties on the buns and top with lettuce, tomato, and onion.

6. Serve and enjoy.

Baked Sweet Potato Fries

Ingredients:

- 2 peeled and thinly sliced sweet potatoes

- 2 tablespoons olive oil

- 1/2 teaspoon garlic powder

- 1/2 teaspoon paprika

- Salt and pepper, to taste

Method:

1. Preheat the oven to 400°F.

2. Place parchment paper on a baking pan.

3. Place the sweet potato strips on the baking sheet and drizzle with olive oil.

4. Sprinkle with garlic powder, paprika, salt, and pepper.

5. Bake for 20-25 minutes, until golden brown and crispy

6. Serve and enjoy.

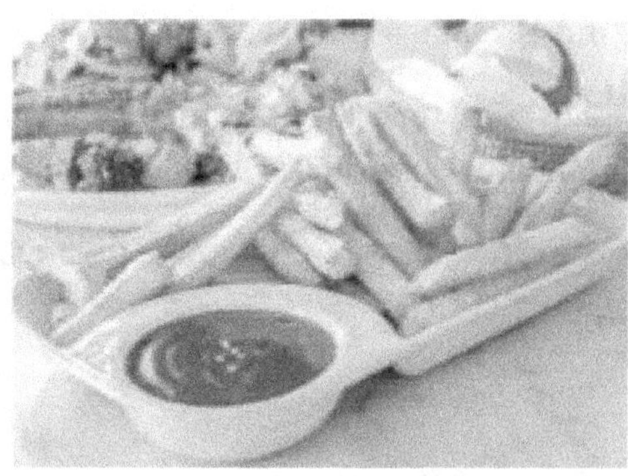

Grilled Zucchini and Summer Squash

Ingredients:

- 2 zucchini, sliced into 1/4-inch thick slices

- 2 summer squash, sliced into 1/4-inch thick slices

- 2 tablespoons olive oil

- 2 cloves garlic, minced

- 1/2 teaspoon dried oregano

- Salt and pepper, to taste

Method:

1. Preheat the grill to medium-high heat.

2. In a large bowl, combine the zucchini, summer squash, olive oil, garlic, oregano, salt, and pepper.

3. Toss to combine.

4. Place the vegetables on the preheated grill and cook for 4-5 minutes per side, until softened and lightly charred.

5. Serve and enjoy.

Turkey Taco Lettuce Wraps

Ingredients:

- 1 pound ground turkey

- 1 tablespoon chili powder

- 1 teaspoon garlic powder

- 1 teaspoon cumin

- 2 tablespoons tomato paste

- Salt and pepper, to taste

- 1 head iceberg lettuce, leaves separated

- 2 tomatoes, diced

- 1/2 cup shredded cheese

- 1/4 cup reduced-sodium salsa

Method:

1. Melt butter in a big saucepan on a high heat

2. Add the ground turkey and cook for 3-4 minutes, until no longer pink.

3. Add the chili powder, garlic powder, cumin, tomato paste, salt, and pepper.

4. Cook for an additional 3-4 minutes, until everything is cooked through.

5. Pile the lettuce leaves with the turkey mixture and top with tomatoes, cheese, and salsa.

6. Serve and enjoy.

Grilled Eggplant Parmesan

Ingredients:

- 2 eggplants, sliced into 1/2-inch thick rounds

- 2 tablespoons olive oil

- 1/2 teaspoon garlic powder

- Salt and pepper, to taste

- 1 cup marinara sauce

- 1 cup shredded mozzarella cheese

- 2 tablespoons chopped fresh basil

Method:

1. Preheat the grill to medium-high heat.

2. In a large bowl, combine the eggplant, olive oil, garlic powder, salt, and pepper.

3. Toss to combine.

4. Place the eggplant on the preheated grill and cook for 4-5 minutes per side, until softened and lightly charred.

5. Remove the eggplant from the grill and place on a baking sheet.

6. Top with marinara sauce, mozzarella cheese, and basil.

7. Bake for 10 minutes, until the cheese is melted and bubbly.

8. Serve and enjoy.

Baked Chicken with Apples and Pecans

Ingredients:

- 4 boneless, skinless chicken breasts

-2 tablespoons olive oil

- 2 tablespoons Dijon mustard

- 2 apples, cored and sliced

- 1/2 cup chopped pecans

- 2 tablespoons honey

- Salt and pepper, to taste

Method:

1. Preheat the oven to 400°F.

2. Line an oven sheet with foil and gently grease with cooking spray.

3. Place the chicken breasts on the baking sheet and brush with olive oil and Dijon mustard.

4. Top with apples, pecans, honey, salt, and pepper.

5. Bake for 20-25 minutes, until the chicken is cooked through.

6. Serve and enjoy.

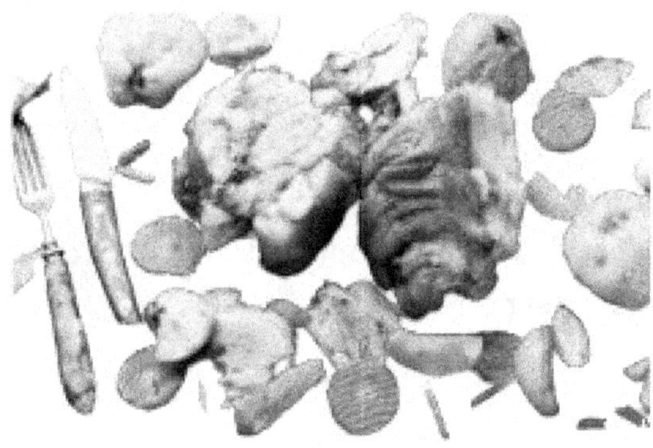

Baked Chicken with Apples and Pecans

Asparagus and Mushroom Quinoa

Ingredients:

- 1 cup uncooked quinoa

- 2 tablespoons olive oil

- 1 cup sliced mushrooms

- 1 cup chopped asparagus

- 2 cloves garlic, minced

- 2 tablespoons balsamic vinegar

- Salt and pepper, to taste

Method:

1. Cook the quinoa according to package directions.

2. In a big skillet with a medium-high temperature, heat the olive oil.

3. Add the mushrooms and asparagus and cook for 3-4 minutes, until softened.

4. Cook for 1-2 minutes after adding the garlic.

5. Stir in the cooked quinoa and balsamic vinegar and season with salt and pepper.

6. Continue to cook for another 2-3 minutes, or until everything is thoroughly heated.

7. Serve and enjoy.

Greek Yogurt Chicken Salad

Ingredients:

- 2 cups cooked, shredded chicken

- 1 cup plain Greek yogurt

- 1/4 cup chopped red onion

- 1/4 cup chopped celery

- 1/4 cup raisins

- 1 tablespoon lemon juice

- Salt and pepper, to taste

Method:

1. In a large bowl, combine the chicken, Greek yogurt, red onion, celery, and raisins.

2. Season with salt and pepper and drizzle with lemon juice.

3. Toss to combine.

4. Serve with lettuce or on a sandwich.

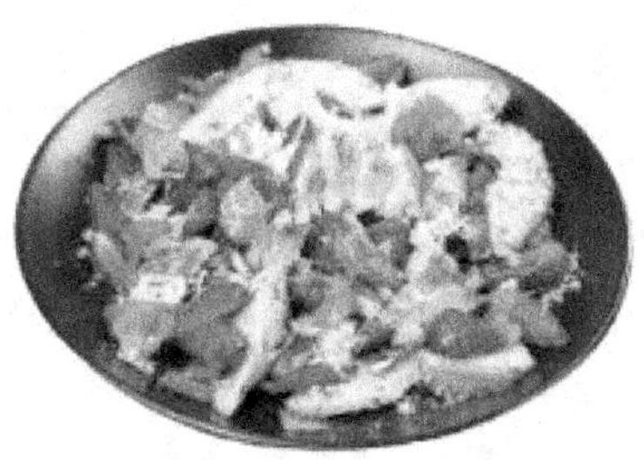

Greek Yogurt Chicken Salad

Spicy Chickpea and Kale Salad

Ingredients:

- 2 cups cooked chickpeas

- 2 cups chopped kale

- 1/4 cup diced red onion

- 2 tablespoons olive oil

- 2 tablespoons lemon juice

- 1 teaspoon cumin

- 1 teaspoon chili powder

- Salt and pepper, to taste

Method:

1. In a large bowl, combine the chickpeas, kale, and red onion.

2. Drizzle with olive oil and lemon juice and season with cumin, chili powder, salt, and pepper.

3. Toss to combine.

4. Serve and enjoy.

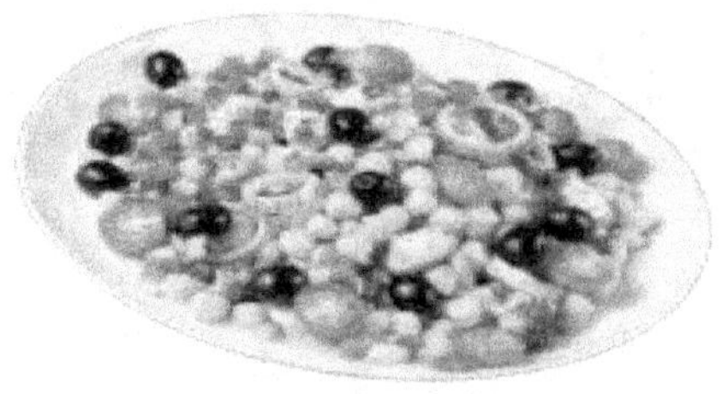

Baked Tilapia with Tomatoes and Olives

Ingredients:

- 4 (4-ounce) tilapia fillets

- 2 tablespoons olive oil

- 2 cloves garlic, minced

- 2 tomatoes, diced

- 1/4 cup sliced olives

- 2 tablespoons capers

- 1 tablespoon lemon juice

- Salt and pepper, to taste

Method:

1. Preheat the oven to 400°F.

2. Line an oven sheet with foil and gently grease with cooking spray.

3. Place the tilapia fillets on the baking sheet and brush with olive oil.

4. Top with garlic, tomatoes, olives, capers, lemon juice, salt, and pepper.

5. Bake for 15-20 minutes, until the tilapia is cooked through.

6. Serve and enjoy.

Steamed Broccoli with Garlic and Soy Sauce

Ingredients:

- 1 head broccoli, cut into florets

- 2 tablespoons olive oil

- 2 cloves garlic, minced

- 2 tablespoons reduced-sodium soy sauce

- 1 tablespoon sesame oil

- Salt and pepper, to taste

Method:

1. Place the broccoli in a steamer basket and steam for 5-7 minutes, until softened and bright green.

2. Warm the olive oil in a large pan over medium flame.

3. Add the garlic in to the skillet and cook for about 1-2 minutes, until fragrant.

4. Add the steamed broccoli and soy sauce and cook for an additional 2-3 minutes.

5. Season with salt and pepper and drizzle with sesame oil.

6. Serve and enjoy.

CHAPTER 6

Dinner Recipes Preparation

Baked Salmon with Roasted Asparagus:

Ingredients:

-4 salmon fillets

-2 tablespoons olive oil

-Salt and pepper, to taste

-1 bunch asparagus

-2 tablespoons lemon juice

Method:

Preheat oven to 350°F. Place salmon fillets in a lightly greased baking dish. Brush with olive oil and season with salt and pepper to taste.

Bake for 15 minutes. Meanwhile, prepare asparagus by tossing with olive oil, salt, and pepper. Put on a baking sheet and roast for 10 minutes in the oven. Plate the salmon and asparagus and drizzle with lemon juice. Enjoy!

Grilled Chicken with Quinoa Pilaf:

Ingredients:

-4 boneless, skinless chicken breasts

-2 tablespoons olive oil

-Salt and pepper, to taste

-1/2 cup quinoa

-1 cup vegetable broth

-1/2 cup diced tomatoes

-1/2 cup diced red onion

-1/4 cup diced bell pepper

-1 tablespoon minced garlic

-2 tablespoons fresh chopped parsley

Method:

Heat a grill to medium-high heat. Drizzle the chicken with olive oil and season with salt and pepper to taste. Grill chicken for 10 minutes, flipping occasionally until cooked through. While chicken is grilling, prepare quinoa pilaf.

Heat a large skillet over medium heat and add the quinoa, broth, tomatoes, red onion, bell pepper, garlic, and parsley. Cook for 8-10 minutes, stirring occasionally until quinoa is cooked through. Plate chicken with quinoa pilaf and enjoy!

Zucchini Noodles with Avocado Sauce:

Ingredients:

-2 medium zucchinis

-2 tablespoons olive oil

-Salt and pepper, to taste

-1 ripe avocado

-2 tablespoons lemon juice

-1/4 cup plain Greek yogurt

Method:

Use a spiralizer to make zucchini noodles. Heat a large skillet over medium heat and add olive oil. Add zucchini noodles to the pan and season lightly with salt and pepper. Cook for 4-5 minutes, stirring occasionally until zucchini noodles are just tender. Meanwhile, prepare avocado sauce by combining avocado, lemon juice, Greek yogurt, and a pinch of salt and pepper in a blender. Blend until smooth.

Plate the zucchini noodles and top with avocado sauce. Enjoy!

Grilled Eggplant Stacks:

Ingredients:

-2 large eggplants

-2 tablespoons olive oil

-Salt and pepper, to taste

-2 tablespoons balsamic vinegar

-1/4 cup ricotta cheese

-1/4 cup tomato sauce

-1/4 cup shredded mozzarella cheese

Method:

Preheat grill to medium-high heat. Slice eggplant into 1/2 inch slices and brush each side with olive oil. Season lightly with salt and pepper. Grill eggplant for 4-5 minutes on each side. Meanwhile, in a small bowl combine balsamic vinegar, ricotta cheese, and a pinch of salt and pepper.

To assemble the eggplant stacks, layer a slice of grilled eggplant with a spoonful of ricotta cheese mixture and a spoonful of tomato sauce.

Top with another slice of grilled eggplant and repeat. Top with shredded mozzarella cheese and place on preheated grill for 4-5 minutes or until cheese is melted and bubbly. Enjoy!

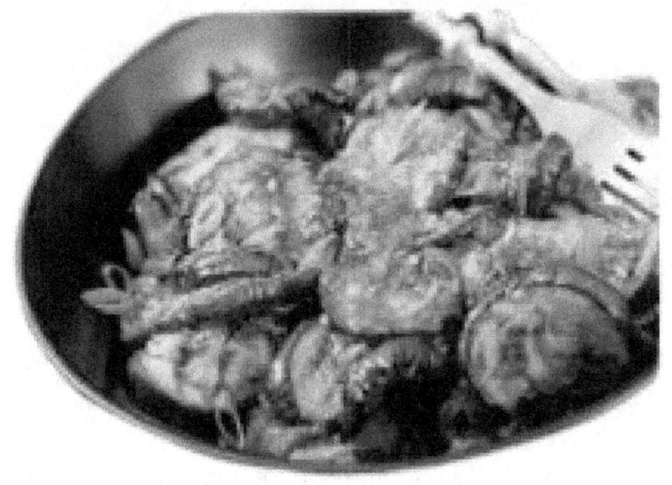

Grilled Eggplant Stacks

Baked Greek Cod:

Ingredients:

-4 cod fillets

-2 tablespoons olive oil

-Salt and pepper, to taste

-1/2 cup diced tomatoes

-1/2 cup diced cucumber

-1/4 cup diced red onion

-1/4 cup Kalamata olives

-2 tablespoons chopped fresh dill

-1 tablespoon minced garlic

-1/4 cup crumbled feta cheese

Method:

Put the steaks in a baking dish that has been gently oiled. Drizzle with olive oil and add pepper and salt to taste. Bake for 15 minutes in the oven. Meanwhile, combine tomatoes, cucumber, onion, olives, dill, garlic, and feta cheese in a medium mixing bowl.

After 15 minutes, top each fish fillet with the tomato mixture. Heat for another 5 minutes, or until the fish is cooked thoroughly. Serve and enjoy!

Eggplant Parmesan:

Ingredients:

-1 large eggplant

-2 tablespoons olive oil

-Salt and pepper, to taste

-1/4 cup tomato sauce

-1/4 cup grated Parmesan cheese

-1/4 cup shredded mozzarella cheese

Method:

Preheat oven to 375°F. Slice eggplant into 1/4 inch slices and brush each side with olive oil. Season lightly with salt and pepper. Place eggplant slices on a baking sheet and roast in the oven for 10 minutes. Flip eggplant slices and bake for an additional 10 minutes.

Remove eggplant from oven and top each slice with a spoonful of tomato sauce, Parmesan cheese, and mozzarella cheese. Put the fish fillets in a baking dish that has been gently oiled. Heat for another 10 minutes, or until the cheese is melted and bubbling. Enjoy!

Baked Teriyaki Tofu:

Ingredients:

-1 block firm tofu

-2 tablespoons olive oil

-Salt and pepper, to taste

-1/4 cup teriyaki sauce

-1/4 cup diced bell pepper

-1/4 cup diced red onion

-1 tablespoon minced garlic

Method:

Preheat oven to 375°F. Drain tofu and cut into cubes. Place tofu cubes in a lightly greased baking dish and brush with olive oil. Season lightly with salt and pepper. Bake for 20 minutes, stirring occasionally.

Meanwhile, in a small bowl, combine teriyaki sauce, bell pepper, onion, and garlic.

After tofu has baked for 20 minutes, pour teriyaki mixture over the tofu and stir to combine. Bake for an additional 10 minutes or until tofu is cooked through. Enjoy!

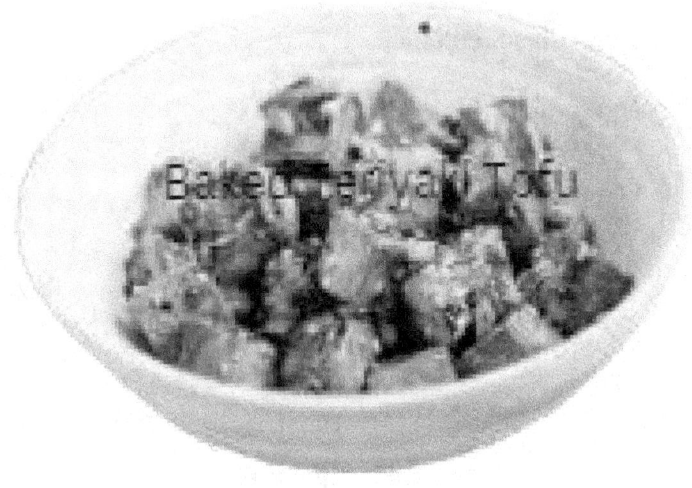

Baked Teriyaki Tofu

Roasted Vegetable Quinoa Bowls:

Ingredients:

-1/2 cup quinoa

-1 cup vegetable broth

-1/2 cup diced bell pepper

-1/2 cup diced zucchini

-1/2 cup diced red onion

-2 tablespoons olive oil

-Salt and pepper, to taste

-1/4 cup crumbled feta cheese

Method:

Preheat oven to 375°F. Heat a large skillet over medium heat and add quinoa and vegetable broth. Bring to a boil, reduce heat, and simmer for 10 minutes until quinoa is cooked through.

Meanwhile, in a medium bowl combine bell pepper, zucchini, onion, olive oil, and a pinch of salt and pepper.

Place vegetables on a baking sheet and roast in the oven for 10 minutes.

Divide quinoa among 4 bowls and top with roasted vegetables. Sprinkle each bowl with feta cheese and enjoy!

Roasted Garlic and Whit Bean Soup:

Ingredients:

-2 tablespoons olive oil

-1 head garlic

-Salt and pepper, to taste

-1 large onion, diced

-3 stalks celery, diced

-2 carrots, diced

-4 cups vegetable broth

-2 cans white beans, drained and rinsed

-1 teaspoon dried thyme

-1/4 cup chopped fresh parsley

Method:

Preheat oven to 375°F. Cut top off garlic head and brush with olive oil. Sprinkle with salt and pepper. Wrap garlic head in foil and bake for 30 minutes. Heat a large pot over medium heat and add olive oil, onion, celery, and carrots. Season lightly with salt and pepper and cook for 5 minutes, stirring occasionally.

Add vegetable broth, beans, thyme, and parsley to the pot and bring to a boil. Reduce heat and simmer for 10 minutes. Squeeze roasted garlic cloves into the pot and stir to combine. Simmer for an additional 5 minutes. Serve warm and enjoy!

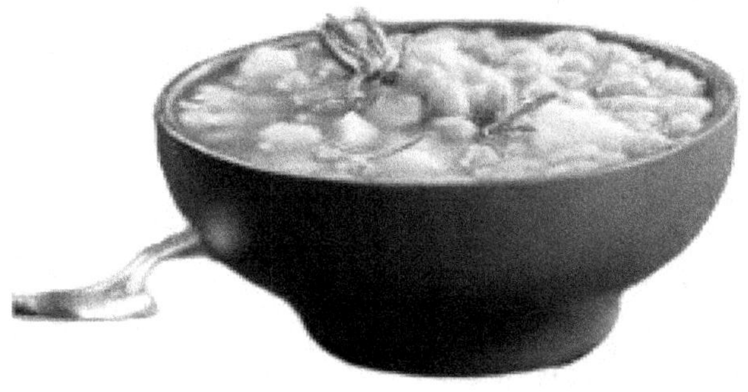

Roasted Garlic and Whit Bean Soup

Baked Tempeh with Orange Sauce:

Ingredients:

-1 package tempeh

-2 tablespoons olive oil

-Salt and pepper, to taste

-1/4 cup orange juice

-1 tablespoon honey

-1 tablespoon white wine vinegar

-1 teaspoon minced garlic

-1/4 teaspoon ground ginger

Method:

Preheat oven to 375°F. Cut tempeh into cubes and place in a lightly greased baking dish. Drizzle with olive oil and add some pepper and salt to taste. Bake for 15 minutes, stirring occasionally.

Meanwhile, in a small saucepan combine orange juice, honey, white wine vinegar, garlic, and ginger. Bring to a boil, then lower to a low heat and continue to cook for 5 minutes. After tempeh has baked for 15 minutes, pour orange sauce over the tempeh and stir to combine. Bake for an additional 10 minutes or until tempeh is cooked through. Enjoy!

Broiled Tilapia with Pesto Sauce:

Ingredients:

-4 tilapia fillets

-2 tablespoons olive oil

-Salt and pepper, to taste

-1/4 cup prepared pesto

-1 lemon, sliced

-2 tablespoons fresh chopped parsley

Method:

Preheat broiler. Drizzle tilapia fillets with olive oil on a lightly oiled baking dish. Season lightly with salt and pepper. Broil for 10 minutes, turning halfway through.

Meanwhile, in a small bowl combine pesto and a pinch of salt and pepper.

After tilapia has cooked for 10 minutes, top each fillet with pesto sauce. Place lemon slices on top and broil for an additional 5 minutes or until fish is cooked through. Garnish with parsley and enjoy!

Grilled Vegetable and Hummus Wraps:

Ingredients:

-4 whole wheat tortillas

-1/2 cup prepared hummus

-1/2 cup diced bell pepper

-1/2 cup diced red onion

-1/2 cup diced zucchini

-2 tablespoons olive oil

-Salt and pepper, to taste

Method:

Heat a grill to medium-high heat. In a medium bowl combine bell pepper, onion, zucchini, olive oil, and a pinch of salt and pepper. Toss to combine and place vegetables on preheated grill. Grill for 4-5 minutes, flipping occasionally until vegetables are tender.

To assemble wraps, spread each tortilla with hummus. Top with grilled vegetables and roll up. Enjoy!

Baked Salmon with Mango Salsa:

Ingredients:

-4 salmon fillets

-2 tablespoons olive oil

-Salt and pepper, to taste

-1 cup diced mango

-1/4 cup diced red onion

-1/4 cup diced red bell pepper

-2 tablespoons chopped fresh cilantro

-2 tablespoons lime juice

Method:

Preheat oven to 375°F. Place salmon fillets in a lightly greased baking dish. Brush with olive oil and sprinkle with pepper and salt to taste. Bake for 15 minutes in the oven. Meanwhile, combine mango, onion, bell pepper, cilantro, and lime juice in a medium mixing bowl.

After salmon has baked for 15 minutes, top each fillet with mango salsa. Bake for an additional 5 minutes or until salmon is cooked through. Plate and enjoy!

Grilled Tofu and Vegetable Skewers:

Ingredients:

-1 block firm tofu

-2 tablespoons olive oil

-Salt and pepper, to taste

-1 bell pepper, diced

-1 red onion, diced

-1 zucchini, diced

-1/4 cup teriyaki sauce

Method:

Heat a grill to medium-high heat. Drain tofu and cut into cubes. Place tofu cubes in a shallow bowl and brush with olive oil. Season lightly with salt and pepper. Thread tofu onto skewers with bell pepper, onion, and zucchini.

Grill skewers for 10 minutes, flipping occasionally. Brush with teriyaki sauce and grill for an additional 5 minutes or until tofu is cooked through. Enjoy!

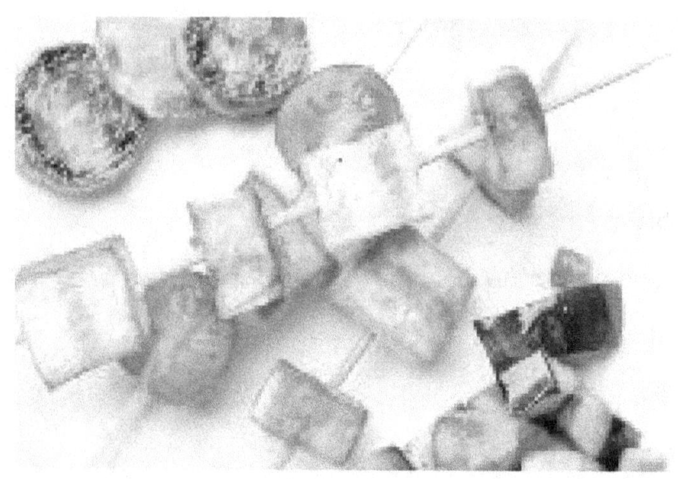

Grilled Tofu and Vegetable Skewers

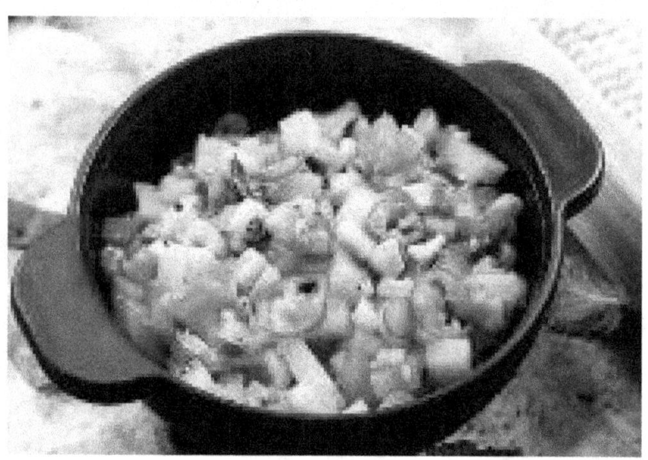

Baked Salmon with Mango Salsa

CHAPTER 7

Snack and Appetizer Recipes

Cucumber and Avocado Salad

Ingredients:

-1 cucumber, peeled and sliced

-1 avocado, peeled and sliced

-1/4 cup fresh cilantro, finely chopped

-1 tablespoons fresh lime juice

-Salt and pepper, to taste

-1 tablespoon olive oil

Method of Preparation:

1. In a medium bowl, combine cucumber slices, avocado slices, and cilantro.

2. Squeeze lime juice over the top and toss gently.

3. Season with salt and pepper, to taste.

4. Drizzle with olive oil and toss gently.

5. Serve chilled.

Zucchini Fritters

Ingredients:

-2 zucchini, grated

-1/4 cup whole wheat flour

-1 egg, lightly beaten

-1/4 teaspoon garlic powder

-Salt and pepper, to taste

-1/4 cup olive oil

Method of Preparation:

1. In a medium bowl, combine grated zucchini, flour, egg, garlic powder, and salt and pepper.

2. In a big pan over medium heat, heat the olive oil.

3. Drop spoonful of the zucchini mixture into the hot oil and cook for 3-4 minutes per side or until golden brown.

4. Take the fritters from the pan and place them on paper towels to drain.

5. Serve warm.

Spinach and Pecan Dip

Ingredients:

-1/2 cup pecans, chopped

-2 cups fresh spinach, chopped

-1/4 cup plain Greek yogurt

-1/4 cup feta cheese

-1 tablespoon olive oil

-Salt and pepper, to taste

Method of Preparation:

1. In a food processor, combine pecans, spinach, yogurt, and feta cheese.

2. Pulse until ingredients are mixed but still have texture.

3. Add olive oil and pulse until combined.

4. Season with salt and pepper, to taste.

5. Serve with crackers or vegetables.

Zucchini and Carrot Noodle Salad

Ingredients:

-2 zucchini, spiralized

-2 carrots, spiralized

-1/4 cup fresh parsley, finely chopped

-1/4 cup olive oil

-1/4 cup lemon juice

-Salt and pepper, to taste

Method of Preparation:

1. In a large bowl, combine spiralized zucchini and carrots.

2. Add parsley, olive oil, and lemon juice and toss to combine.

3. Season with salt and pepper, to taste.

4. Serve chilled.

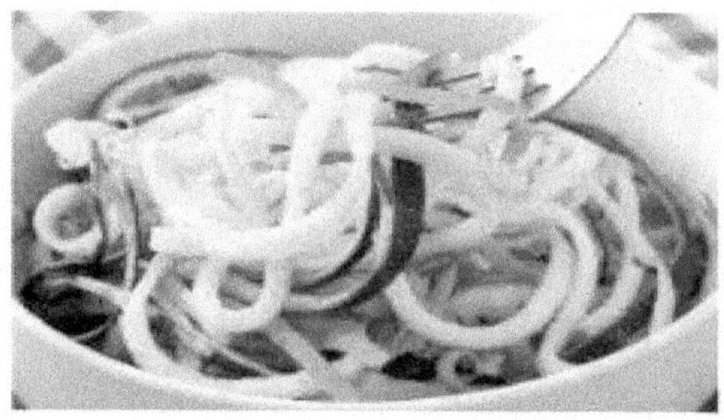

Zucchini and Carrot Noodle Salad

Caprese Salad Skewers

Ingredients:

-2 tomatoes, diced

-1/2 cup fresh mozzarella, diced

-1/4 cup fresh basil, finely chopped

-1 tablespoon olive oil

-Salt and pepper, to taste

-10 wooden skewers

Method of Preparation:

1. In water for 30 minute soak the wooden skewers.

2. In a medium bowl, combine tomatoes, mozzarella, and basil.

3. Sprinkle with olive oil and season to taste with salt and pepper.

4. Thread tomato, mozzarella, and basil onto skewers.

5. Serve chilled.

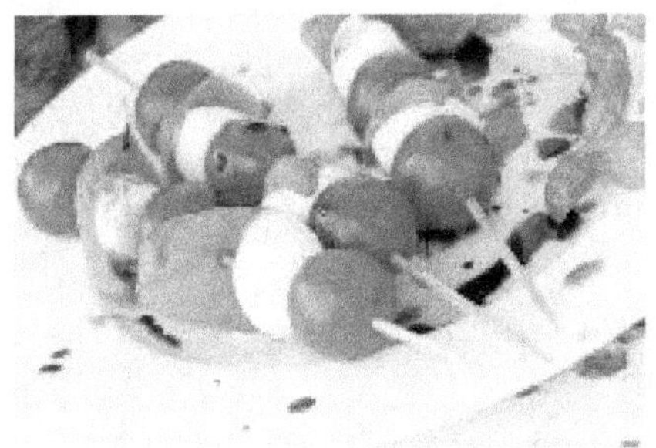

No-Bake Granola Bars

Ingredients:

-2 cups rolled oats

-1/4 cup honey

-1/4 cup peanut butter

-1/4 cup chopped walnuts

-1/4 cup dried cranberries

-1/4 cup chocolate chips

Method of Preparation:

1. In a medium bowl, combine oats, honey, and peanut butter.

2. Stir until ingredients are combined.

3. Mix in walnuts, cranberries, and chocolate chips.

4. Using parchment paper, line a 9"x9" baking sheet.

5. Press granola mixture into the pan and spread evenly.

6. Refrigerate for 1 hour or until set.

7. Cut into bars and serve.

Baked Zucchini Chips

Ingredients:

-2 zucchini, sliced

-1 tablespoon olive oil

-1teaspoon garlic powder

-1/2 teaspoon paprika

-Salt and pepper, to taste

Method of Preparation:

1. Preheat oven to 350°F.

2. Line a baking sheet with parchment paper.

3. Place zucchini slices on parchment paper and brush with olive oil.

4. Season with garlic powder, paprika, salt, and pepper.

5. Bake for 20-25 minutes, flipping once halfway through, or until chips are golden brown and crispy.

6. Serve warm.

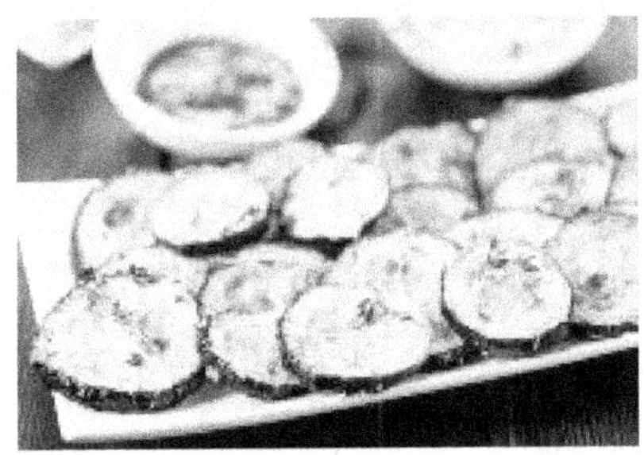

Roasted Red Pepper Hummus

Ingredients:

-1 can chickpeas, drained and rinsed

-1 roasted red pepper, chopped

-2 tablespoons olive oil

-2 tablespoons lemon juice

-1 teaspoon garlic powder

-Salt and pepper, to taste

Method of Preparation:

1. In a food processor, combine chickpeas, roasted red pepper, olive oil, lemon juice, and garlic powder.

2. Pulse until ingredients are combined and hummus is desired consistency.

3. Season with salt and pepper, to taste.

4. Serve with crackers or vegetables.

CHAPTER 8

Vegetable and Side Dish Recipes

Roasted Broccoli

Ingredients:

-1 head of broccoli

-1 tablespoon of olive oil

-Salt and pepper to taste

Method of Preparation:

1. Preheat oven to 400 degrees F.

2. Cut the broccoli into florets and spread onto a baking sheet.

3. Season the broccoli with salt and pepper and drizzle with olive oil.

4. Roast in the oven for 15-20 minutes, or until the broccoli is tender and lightly browned.

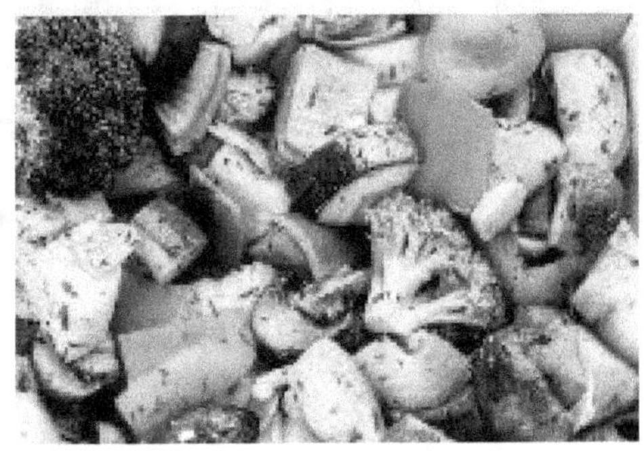

Roasted Cauliflower

Ingredients:

-1 head of cauliflower

-1 tablespoon of olive oil

-Salt and pepper to taste

Method of Preparation:

1. Preheat oven to 400 degrees F.

2. Spread the cauliflower florets out on a baking pan.

3. Season the cauliflower with salt and pepper and drizzle with olive oil.

4. Roast in the oven for 15-20 minutes, or until the cauliflower is tender and lightly browned.

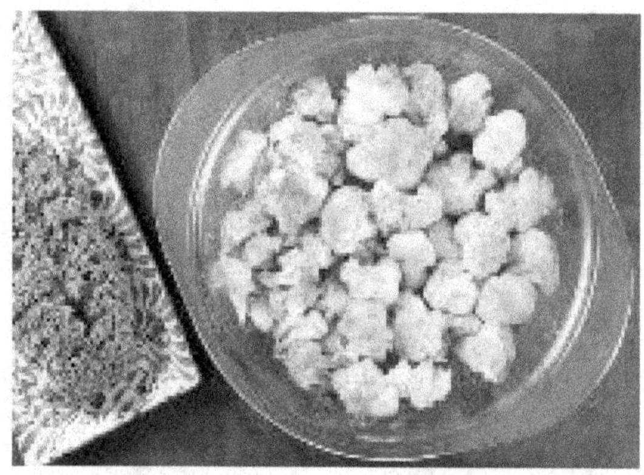

Baked Apples

Ingredients:

-4 apples

-1 tablespoon of olive oil

-Ground cinnamon to taste

Method of Preparation:

1. Preheat oven to 375 degrees F.

2. Cut the apples in half and core.

3. Drizzle the olive oil over the apples and sprinkle with cinnamon.

4. Bake in the oven for 30-35 minutes, or until the apples are tender and lightly browned.

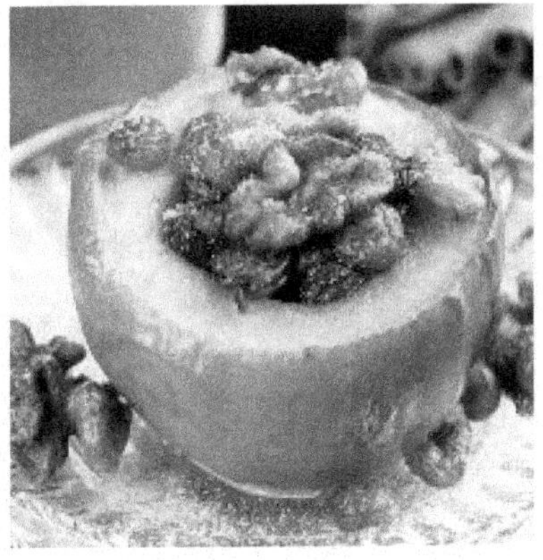

Baked Carrots

Ingredients:

-4 carrots

-1 tablespoon of olive oil

-Salt and pepper to taste

Method of Preparation:

1. Preheat oven to 400 degrees F.

2. Cut the carrots into slices and spread onto a baking sheet.

3. Drizzle the olive oil over the carrots and season with salt and pepper.

4. Bake in the oven for 15-20 minutes, or until the carrots are tender and lightly browned.

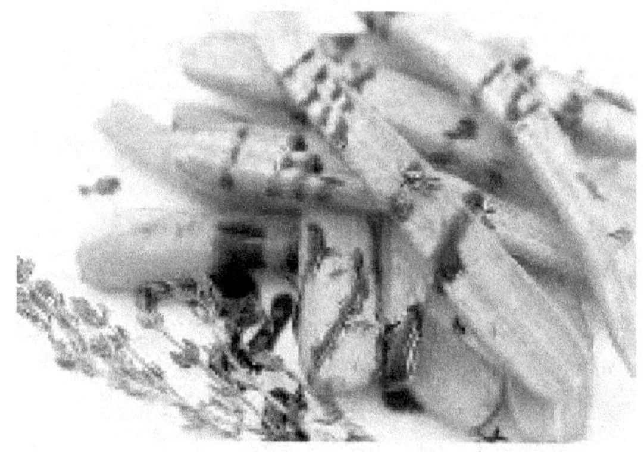

Roasted Red Peppers

Ingredients:

-4 red peppers

-1 tablespoon of olive oil

-Salt and pepper to taste

Method of Preparation:

1. Preheat oven to 400 degrees F.

2. Cut the peppers into slices and spread onto a baking sheet.

3. Drizzle the olive oil over the peppers and season with salt and pepper.

4. Roast in the oven for 15-20 minutes, or until the peppers are tender and lightly browned.

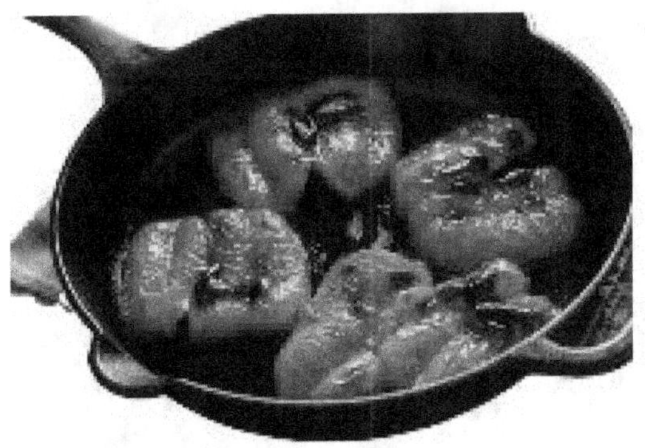

Baked Butternut Squash

Ingredients:

-1 butternut squash

-1 tablespoon of olive oil

-Salt and pepper to taste

Method of Preparation:

1. Preheat oven to 400 degrees F.

2. Scoop out the seeds after cutting the squash in half.

3. Drizzle the olive oil over the squash and season with salt and pepper.

4. Bake in the oven for 30-35 minutes, or until the squash is tender and lightly browned.

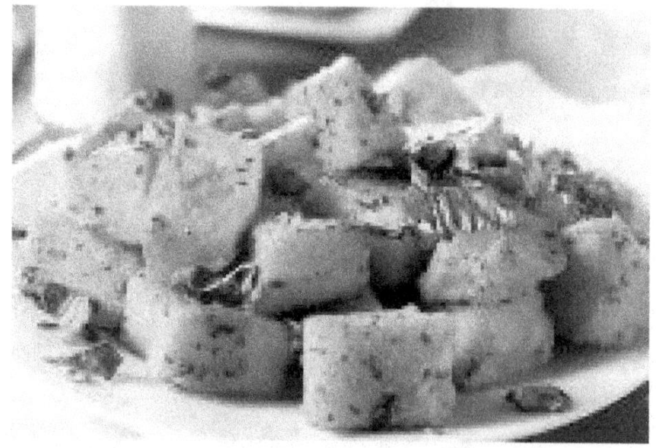

CHAPTER 9

Dessert Recipes with method of preparation

Banana Oatmeal Smoothie

Ingredients:

-1/2 banana

-1/2 cup oats

-1/2 cup almond milk

-1 teaspoon honey

-1/4 teaspoon cinnamon

-1/4 teaspoon vanilla extract

Method of Preparation:

1. Combine all of the ingredients in a blender and blend everything together until smooth.

2. Pour into a glass and serve

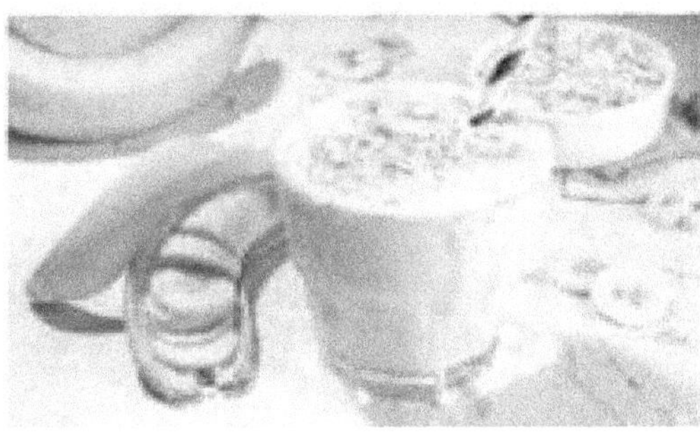

Apple Pie Parfait

Ingredients:

-1/2 cup diced apples

-1 tablespoon rolled oats

-1 tablespoon honey

-1/4 teaspoon cinnamon

-1/4 teaspoon nutmeg

-1/2 cup plain Greek yogurt

Method of Preparation:

1. In a bowl, combine the diced apples, rolled oats, honey, cinnamon, and nutmeg.

2. In a glass, layer the apple mixture and Greek yogurt.

3. Repeat until the glass is full and enjoy.

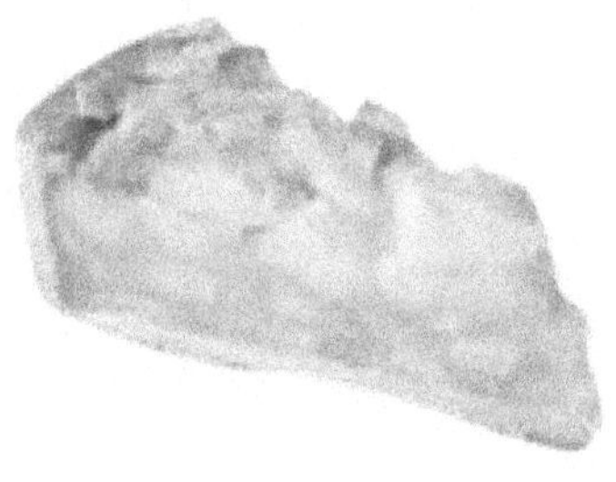

Apple Pie Parfait

Avocado Chocolate Mousse

Ingredients:

-1 medium avocado

-2 tablespoons cocoa powder

-2 teaspoons honey

-1/4 teaspoon vanilla extract

-1/4 teaspoon almond

Method of Preparation:

1. Mash the avocado until smooth.

2. Add the cocoa powder, honey, vanilla extract, and almond and mix until fully combined.

3. Spoon the mixture into a bowl and enjoy.

Sweet Potato Brownies

Ingredients:

-1 sweet potato

-1/2 cup cocoa powder

-2 tablespoons honey

-1/4 teaspoon baking soda

-1/4 teaspoon baking powder

Method of Preparation:

1. Preheat the oven to 350 degrees F.

2. Bake the sweet potato for 30 minutes.

3. Once cool, mash the sweet potato and add the cocoa powder, honey, baking soda, and baking powder.

4. Mix until fully combined.

5. Pour the mixture into a greased 8x8 inch baking pan and bake for 25 minutes.

6. Once cool, cut into squares and enjoy.

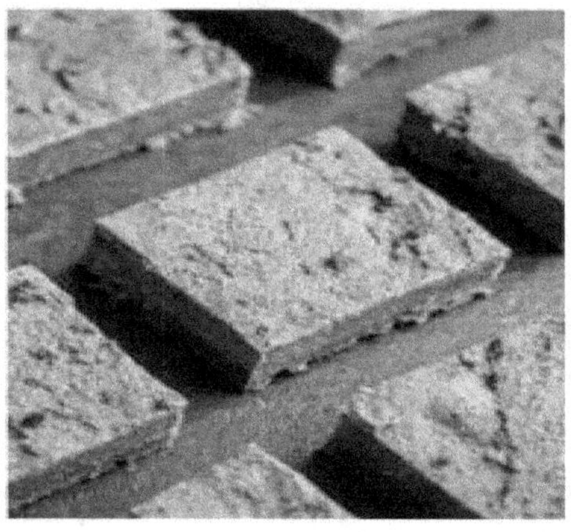

Sweet Potato Brownies

Banana Coconut Bread

Ingredients:

-1 banana

-1/2 cup rolled oats

-1/4 cup coconut flakes

-1/4 cup almond milk

-2 tablespoons honey

-1/4 teaspoon baking

Method of Preparation:

1. Preheat the oven to 350 degrees F.

2. Mash the banana in a basin until smooth.

3. Add the rolled oats, coconut flakes, almond milk, honey, and baking powder.

4. Mix until fully combined.

5. Pour the mixture into a greased 8x8 inch baking pan and bake for 25 minutes.

6. Once cool, cut into slices and enjoy.

Pear Walnut Bread

Ingredients:

-1 pear

-1/2 cup rolled oats

-1/4 cup walnuts

-1/4 cup almond milk

-2 tablespoons honey

-1/4 teaspoon baking powder

Method of Preparation:

1. Preheat the oven to 350 degrees F.

2. Dice the pear and add to a bowl with the rolled oats, walnuts, almond milk, honey, and baking powder.

3. Mix until fully combined.

4. Pour the mixture into a greased 8x8 inch baking pan and bake for 25 minutes.

5. Once cool, cut into slices and enjoy.

Chocolate Banana Bites

Ingredients:

-2 bananas

-2 tablespoons cocoa powder

-2 tablespoons honey

-1/4 teaspoon cinnamon

Method of Preparation:

1. Slice the bananas into thin slices and place on a parchment-lined baking sheet.

2. In a bowl, mix together the cocoa powder, honey, and cinnamon.

3. Brush the mixture onto the banana slices.

4. Bake at 350 degrees F for 20 minutes.

5. Once cool, enjoy.

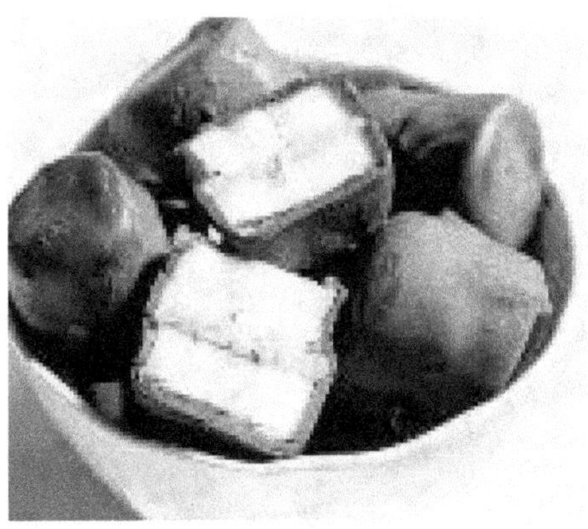

Chocolate Coconut Bites

Ingredients:

-1/2 cup coconut flakes

-1/4 cup cocoa powder

-2 tablespoons honey

-1/4 teaspoon vanilla extract

Method of Preparation:

1. in a bowl, mix together the coconut flakes, cocoa powder, honey, and vanilla extract.

2. Form the mixture into small balls.

3. Place on a parchment-lined baking sheet and bake at 350 degrees F for 20 minutes.

4. Once cool, enjoy.

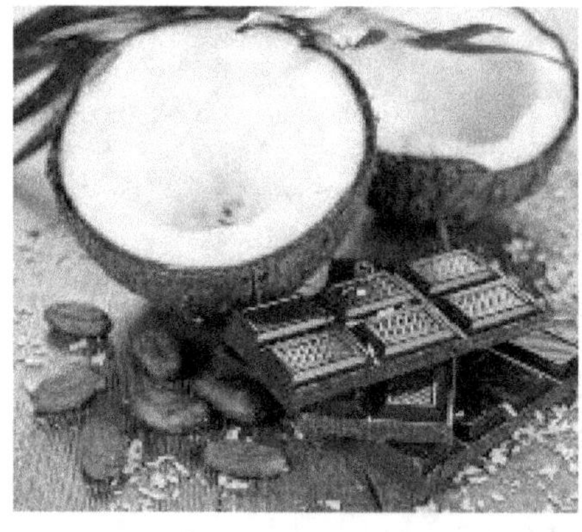

CHAPTER 10

Making the Big Dash Diet Work for You

The Big Dash Diet is an eating plan that focuses on enhancing your overall health by consuming a variety of foods and limiting your consumption of saturated fat and salt.

It encourages you to eat more fruits and vegetables, whole grains, lean proteins, low-fat dairy products like yogurt, and healthy fats like olive oil, canola oil, and nuts. This diet also recommends limiting your intake of processed foods, sweets, and alcohol.

To make the Big Dash Diet work for you, you must be willing to make particular food and lifestyle modifications. Here are some pointers to get you started:

1. Eat meals that are high in nutrients. The Big Dash Diet is based on eating a range of nutrient-dense foods such as fruits, vegetables, whole grains, lean meats, and low-fat dairy products.

Eat a range of colors and fill half your plate with fruits and veggies. Whole grains, such as brown rice and whole-wheat bread, should be preferred over refined grains, such as white bread and white rice. Lean proteins, such as fish, poultry, beans, and lentils, should be preferred over fatty proteins, such as red meat, pig, and processed meats.

2. Minimize your intake of processed meals. Processed foods frequently include high levels of salt, saturated fat, and added sugars. Certain foods should be limited or avoided as much as possible. Instead, prioritize full, unprocessed meals.

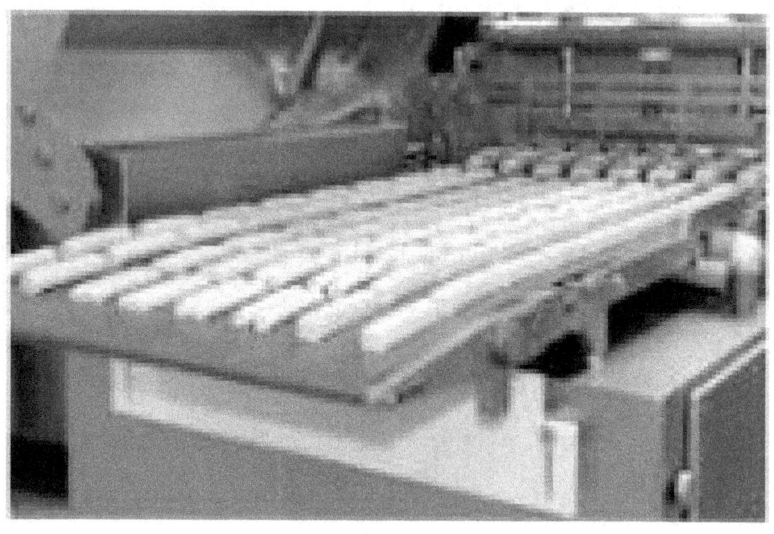

Limit processed foods

3. Consume healthy fats. The Big Dash Diet emphasizes healthy fats including olive oil, canola oil, almonds, and avocado. Good fats can help you feel satisfied for extended periods of time while also providing vital fatty acids, vitamins, and minerals.

4. Keep portion amounts in mind. Even nutritious meals might induce weight gain if consumed in excess. Use smaller dishes and bowls, and measure out single quantities of food to avoid overeating.

5. Start moving. Exercise is an essential component of any healthy eating regimen. Try to get at least 30 minutes of physical activity on most days of the week.

To make the Big Dash Diet work for you, you must be dedicated and committed. You may improve your health by making a few easy modifications to your dietary habits.

For example, if you eat a lot of processed foods like chips and cookies, consider replacing them with healthy choices like fruits, vegetables, whole grains, nuts, and low-fat dairy.

If you don't get much physical activity, try to find activities you love, such as walking, bicycling, swimming, or participating in a sport.

You may make the Big Dash Diet work for you by making a few little adjustments.

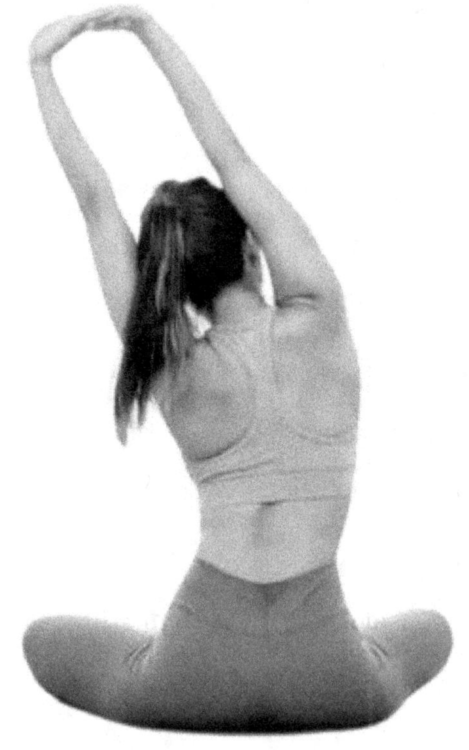

Exercise Regularly

CHAPTER 11

Adapting Low Sodium Recipes to Suit Your Needs

As individuals become more aware of the health advantages of lowering their sodium intake, low sodium meals are becoming more popular. Several dishes are readily adaptable to a low salt diet while still providing tasty and healthy meals. Here are some pointers to help you adjust your favorite recipes to your specific needs:

1. Employ herbs and spices instead of salt: Using tasty herbs and spices instead of salt is one approach to minimize sodium in meals. Instead of salt, consider adding herbs like basil, oregano, rosemary, and garlic powder to foods to add flavor.

2. When shopping for ingredients for a low sodium dish, seek for things labeled "low sodium" or "no added salt." You may also substitute fresh or frozen veggies for canned vegetables, as canned vegetables sometimes include extra salt.

3. Select reduced sodium condiments: Ketchup, mustard, and soy sauce are all rich in sodium. When cooking a low sodium food, choose reduced sodium versions of these condiments or recipes that use natural ingredients such as lemon juice or vinegar instead.

4. Decrease the quantity of salt in a recipe: Certain recipes may ask for a specific amount of salt, but you may reduce it or even leave it out entirely. Add a pinch of salt at a time until you achieve the desired taste.

5. Lemon and lime juice can be used to provide taste without the need of salt. To enhance the flavor of a recipe, try adding a few drops.

These suggestions might help you modify your favorite meals to meet your low sodium requirements. To get the right taste combination for your meals, experiment with different herbs and spices, low sodium items, and condiments.

With a little imagination, you can prepare tasty, healthy meals that are low in salt while remaining flavorful.

For example, if you want to create a favorite pasta meal reduced sodium, focus on lowering the salt level of the components. Make your own spaghetti sauce with tomatoes, onion, garlic, herbs, and a touch of olive oil instead of buying it. You may also use whole wheat pasta, which is lower in salt than normal spaghetti. To end, scatter some freshly chopped herbs and a squeeze of lemon juice on top. This adds a zesty taste without adding salt.

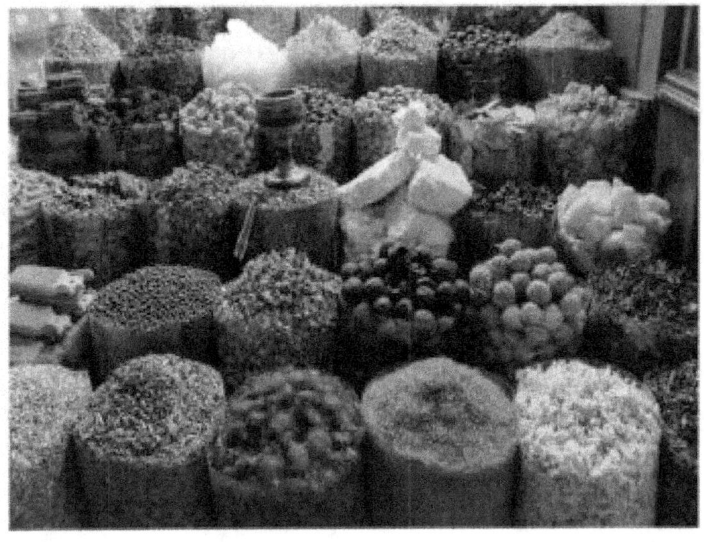

Use herbs and spices

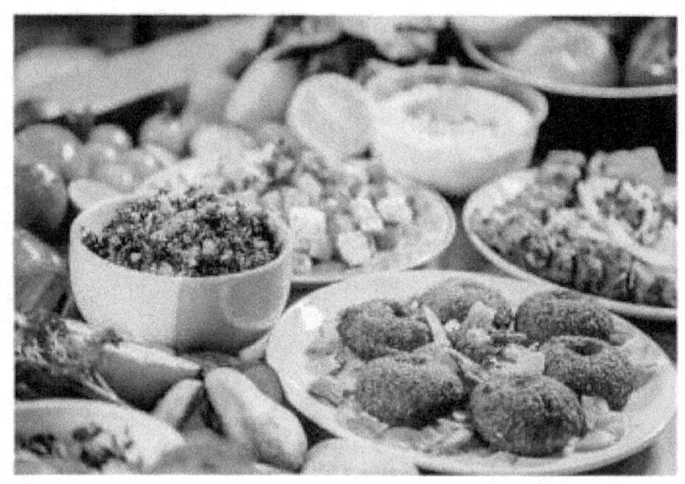

Eat Healthy

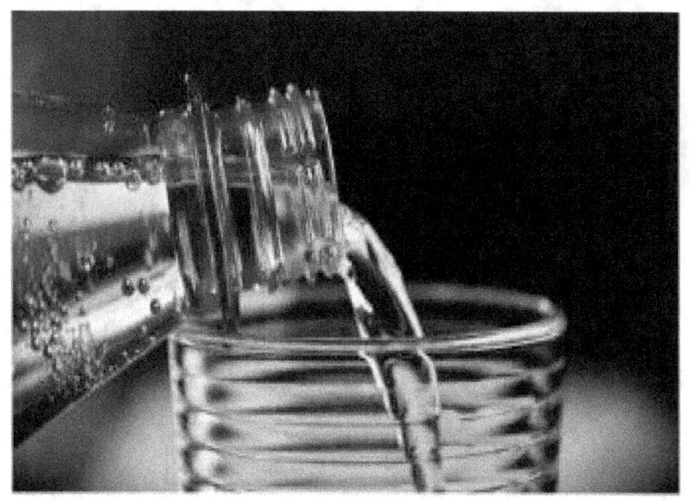

Drink Enough Water

CONCLUSION

Finally, The Big Dash Diet Cookbook for Beginners Low Sodium Recipes is a fantastic resource for anybody trying to enhance their overall health and well-being through a nutritious diet.

These low-sodium dishes, which adhere to the principles of the DASH (Dietary Approaches to Stop Hypertension) diet, give a delicious and gratifying method to lower blood pressure, cut cholesterol, and encourage weight reduction.

This cookbook also stresses fruits and vegetables, whole grains, lean meats, and low-fat dairy products. It offers a holistic approach to healthy eating that may benefit people of different ages and backgrounds.

The Big Dash Diet Cookbook for Beginners is a must-read whether you want to manage your blood pressure, enhance your heart health, or simply eat healthier.

So, why delay? Begin preparing some tasty and nutritious low-sodium meals now and discover how simple and pleasurable healthy eating can be.

You'll be on your road to a better, happier self in no time with the guidance of this cookbook!

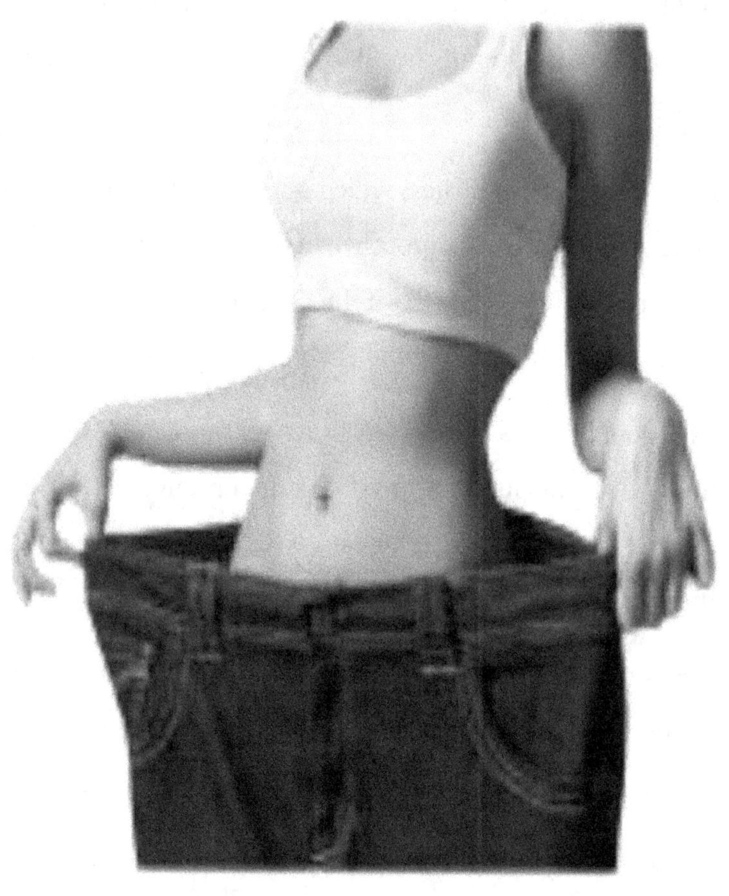